THE WHICH? GUIDE TO
MEN'S HEALTH

GW00320227

About the Author

Dr Steve Carroll MB, BS, MRCS, LRCP is a former GP who now writes full-time on medical and health issues for both consumer and professional publications. Health education is his speciality and he writes regularly for *Which? way to Health* and *Bella* magazines. He is the author of *The Complete Family Guide to Healthy Living* and has contributed to several other health books. Dr Carroll's other main interest is sports medicine: he was previously Assistant Team Doctor for Tottenham Hotspur Football Club and Expedition Doctor for the Ian Botham Hannibal Charity Trek across the Alps.

THE WHICH? GUIDE TO MEN'S HEALTH

DR STEVE CARROLL

WHICH?
BOOKS

CONSUMERS' ASSOCIATION

Which? Books are commissioned and researched by
The Association for Consumer Research and published by
Consumers' Association, 2 Marylebone Road, London NW1 4DF
Distributed by The Penguin Group:
Penguin Books Ltd, 27 Wrights Lane, London W8 5TZ

First edition June 1994

British Library Cataloguing in Publication Data
Carroll, Steve
('Which?' Consumer Guides)
I. Title II. Bezear, Andrew III. Series
613.04233
ISBN 0 85202 545 9

Cover illustrations by ACE/Benelux Press, ACE/Mauritius, ACE/Bill Bachmann
Text illustrations by Andrew Bezear
Typographic design by Paul Saunders
Index by Marie Lorimer

Thanks to Nikki Carroll for help with the production of the manuscript

Typeset by Litho Link Ltd, Welshpool, Powys
Printed and bound by Firmin-Didot (France), Group Herissey,
Nº d'impression: 26796

CONTENTS

INTRODUCTION

Although some men are beginning to take more of an interest in their physical, emotional and sexual well-being, men in general tend to neglect their health. Statistically, a man is only half as likely as a woman to visit the doctor – a difference that cannot be explained just by consultations relating to gynaecology and family planning. A recent MORI poll (July 1992) revealed that 21 per cent of men were either reluctant, or needed encouragement, to go to their GP. Although they might make more fuss over a minor illness – such as a simple cold – they tend to be less willing to visit a doctor to have a symptom diagnosed, even though it may be an early warning of a serious disorder for which prompt treatment could make a huge difference.

Ask a man how he feels and he will invariably say he's fine, regardless of how severely or for how long he has been suffering from a health problem. It is often not until a crisis has occurred and he is on his way to hospital that the true state of his health becomes known. So the impetus to change to a more healthy lifestyle may come only once a man has had a heart attack, for example, and survived.

The problem is that men's health is regarded primarily as the concern of women, who are seen as being responsible not only for their own health but also for the health of their partners and children. Currently, most health information is targeted at women, mainly through magazines, books, TV and radio programmes. The majority of health leaflets are available in health centres and GPs' surgeries – places which men are less likely to frequent. As a result, health advice may not reach men who live alone because they're unmarried, separated or divorced, or men living with a male partner or in a household consisting only of men.

Men are certainly badly informed about many important aspects of their health. The above-mentioned MORI poll showed that, despite the fact that the death rate from prostate disease is four times the mortality rate from cervical cancer and that more than one in three men can expect to suffer from some form of prostate disease before the age of 50, only 32 per cent of men knew anything about their prostate gland.

Very few men have been taught how to examine their own testicles for the warning signs of cancer, yet over 1,000 new cases of testicular cancer are diagnosed each year in the UK – more than half in men under the age of 35. In fact, the number of men developing testicular cancer has doubled over the past 20 years and is expected to double again in the next 20. As this type of cancer can be successfully cured if treated in the early stages, self-examination (described in this book) is a potentially life-saving technique.

And despite all the publicity about HIV and AIDS, the safer sex message does not appear to be influencing sexual behaviour significantly. For example, the incidence of gonorrhoea (a reliable yardstick of safer sex practices), which declined during the 1980s, is once again on the increase.

This book has been written with the aim of providing health advice and information related specifically to the needs of men, as well as encouraging both men *and* their partners to take a more active interest in health issues.

Men – the weaker sex

Women have been described as the weaker sex, but men are twice as likely to die before they reach the age of 65 (usually from preventable conditions such as heart disease, stroke and certain types of cancer). In fact, men have an average life expectancy of just 72 years as against women's 78 years and are twice as likely to commit suicide, which suggests that they tend to neglect their emotional as well as their physical health.

Women's health may be protected by the female sex hormone oestrogen, but even after the menopause – when levels of this hormone plummet – women still have lower death rates from the major killer diseases and are four times more likely to live beyond the age of 85. So why is it that being a man may seriously damage your health?

One major difference between the sexes is that men tend, in general, to have much less healthy lifestyles than women. Men are more likely to smoke, drink too much alcohol, take too little exercise, eat a poor diet and fail to cope effectively with stress – all of which are known to contribute to the development of a variety of serious illnesses. And although men may be aware of the health risks associated with particular habits and behaviour, they may feel more pressure to project a devil-may-care image in public. Some men don't like to be seen ordering healthy food when eating with other men, for example, or may be pressurised by male friends or colleagues at work to drink more alcohol and not to quit smoking.

This book shows how easy it is for you to take control of those factors which might otherwise be undermining your physical, emotional and sexual health – without spoiling your enjoyment of life. To help you appreciate the need to care for your body and what can go wrong with its various components, the book begins with a detailed description of the different body systems and organs. It contains simple, practical advice on how to eat better, take more exercise, give up smoking, cut down on alcohol and control stress levels.

Staying healthy is not only about having a healthy outlook, nor is this book just for those men who fit the stereotype of the overweight smoker slumped in front of the TV with a can of lager and a plate of chips. It advises on protective measures, including immunisation, and explains how to recognise the early-warning symptoms of serious illnesses (and which symptoms to report to the doctor), how to examine different parts of your body yourself and advises on when to attend for screening tests, such as blood pressure and cholesterol measurement.

Following all this advice won't, of course, guarantee you a long life totally free from serious illness, but it will give you a much better chance of staying healthy and enjoying a better quality of life.

Note Addresses and telephone numbers for organisations marked with an asterisk (*) can be found in the address section at the back of the book.

CHAPTER 1

UNDERSTANDING THE MALE BODY

IT IS NOT just doctors, nurses, other medical staff and scientists who need to know about human anatomy and physiology. Everyone should have a basic understanding of the human body and how it works. Such knowledge makes it easier for you to communicate with your doctor, easier to see how an unhealthy lifestyle can damage your body, easier to come to terms with any illness or disease that affects you or someone close to you, and easier to understand why you have developed a particular symptom, why you need a specific investigation and how a drug treatment or surgical operation might help. This chapter also describes how conception occurs in women's bodies.

Heart and circulation

The heart is a powerful muscular pump which beats continuously and rhythmically to force blood into the circulation system. At rest, the normal heart rate may be as low as 50 beats per minute in some men, and as high as 90 beats per minute in others. During strenuous exercise this may increase to about 200 beats per minute.

Situated just to the left of centre of the chest, the heart is approximately the size of a clenched fist. It contains four chambers: two thin-walled upper chambers, called the atria, and two thick-walled lower chambers, called the ventricles. The heart is divided into two by a strong muscular wall, the septum, which prevents the blood flowing through the left atrium and ventricle from mixing with the blood passing through the right atrium and ventricle.

The muscle in the walls of these four chambers consists of a branching network of fibres which will go on contracting spontaneously, rhythmically and completely automatically as long as they are kept supplied with oxygen and nutrients. This type of muscle, known as the myocardium, is not found anywhere else in the body.

A smooth membrane, the endocardium, lines the inside of the heart and is continuous with the lining of the veins and arteries which feed

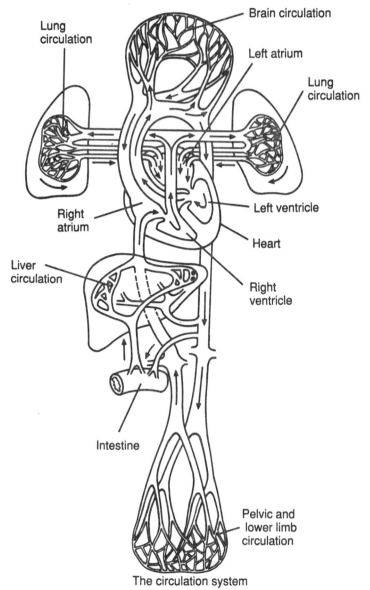

The circulation system

in and out of the heart. A tough, double-layered membranous bag, called the pericardium, surrounds and protects the heart. Between the layers of pericardium is a small amount of lubricating fluid, which allows the heart to expand freely.

How blood circulates

Blood circulates through a complex network of blood vessels in a continuous figure-of-eight circuit, with tiny branches reaching all the cells in the body to ensure they are kept supplied with blood rich in oxygen from the lungs and nutrients from the digestive system.

Oxygen-rich blood leaves the left ventricle through the aorta, which is the largest artery in the body, and is distributed to all organs and tissues through a succession of arterial branches. These arteries become smaller and smaller in diameter, until they feed into tiny vessels known as capillaries.

Oxygen, glucose (sugar) and other nutrients are absorbed into individual cells from the blood passing through nearby capillaries. Carbon dioxide and other waste products are transferred out of the cells. Having given up its oxygen and nutrients, and picked up carbon dioxide and waste products, blood passes from the capillaries into a system of veins. It is the veins that return blood to the heart. Blood returning from the stomach and intestine passes through the liver, which processes nutrients absorbed during digestion.

Two large veins, the superior (upper) vena cava and the inferior (lower) vena cava, return oxygen-depleted blood into the right atrium, from where it is passed down into the right ventricle. When the heart beats, oxygen-depleted blood leaves the right ventricle in the pulmonary artery and is pumped through the lung circulation to be replenished with oxygen. Having taken up oxygen in the lungs, blood returns to the heart in the pulmonary veins, feeding into the left atrium and then down into the left ventricle, ready for the circuit to begin again.

With each heartbeat, blood leaves both sides of the heart simultaneously so there is always some blood being reoxygenated at the same time as the rest is giving up its oxygen. Between each atrium and ventricle, and at the points where the pulmonary artery and aorta leave the heart, there are valves which prevent blood flowing in the wrong direction.

Coronary circulation

To guarantee its own blood supply, the heart has its own exclusive system of arteries, capillaries and veins, known as the coronary circulation. This begins with two arteries emerging from the start of the aorta, branching off to form three main coronary arteries.

Having supplied the heart muscle with oxygen and nutrients from the capillaries, blood is returned to the cardiac veins, which in turn drain into the right atrium.

Respiratory system

This is the system which allows you to breathe oxygen from the air into your lungs and transfer it to the circulation. At the same time, the respiratory system removes excess carbon dioxide from the blood as it passes through the lungs, allowing it to be breathed out.

Air enters the lungs through the upper respiratory tract, which consists of the nose, throat (pharynx) and voice box (larynx). These upper airways feed into the lower respiratory tract, which begins with the windpipe (trachea) and then divides into two large airways known as the bronchi.

The lungs themselves lie on either side of the heart and are cone-shaped. Air passes into each lung through one of the main bronchi, which in turn is able to carry air to and from the whole surface area of that lung by dividing into numerous small branches known as bronchioles.

At the end of each of the smallest bronchioles there are clusters of tiny balloon-like cavities known as alveoli. Over 300 million alveoli cover the entire surface of both lungs. Blood vessels running across each of the alveoli allow for efficient absorption of oxygen from the air coming in, with carbon dioxide passing in the opposite direction out of the bloodstream into the alveoli, to be breathed out.

Breathing mechanism

Breathing is a spontaneous, rhythmical, automatic activity kept going by nerve impulses transmitted from the brain stem at the base of the brain. To breathe in, the muscles between your ribs contract, pulling your rib cage upwards and outwards, and your diaphragm muscle flattens. As a

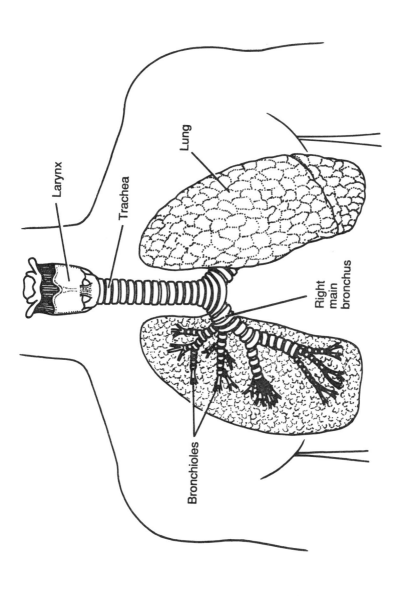

Respiratory system

result of these movements, the chest cavity around the lungs enlarges and the lungs expand to fill the extra space, sucking in air at the same time.

When the rib muscles relax, the rib cage moves back and as the diaphragm relaxes it pushes upwards. Air is thereby squeezed out of the lungs, assisted by their natural elasticity, which encourages them to shrink quickly.

In addition, a lubricating fluid between the two pleural membranes that surround both lungs reduces the amount of friction as they expand and contract.

The normal rate of breathing in an adult man is about 12 breaths per minute, reducing to 9–10 breaths per minute during sleep and increasing to over 20 breaths per minute during vigorous exercise or when under emotional stress.

Purifying the air

Breathing through the nose is healthier than mouth breathing. Not only does the inside of the nose warm up and humidify the air, it also contains tiny hairs which filter out dirt and dust particles.

Other protective mechanisms include the tiny hair-like threads (cilia) lining the insides of the trachea and bronchi, which collect particles found in polluted air, for example, cigarette smoke, preventing them from entering the lungs. There is also a sticky mucus, produced by some of the cells lining the bronchi, which helps trap these impurities.

Coughing is a reflex action which can unblock the airways, for example, shifting a build-up of mucus (sputum). Sneezing is a reflex action that clears particles or excess mucus from the upper respiratory tract.

Digestive system

The digestive system consists of the gastrointestinal tract – a 15-metre-long muscular organ that starts at the mouth and ends at the anus – along with several other important organs which assist with the digestion, absorption and processing of food.

In the first stage of digestion, food is ground up into smaller pieces in the mouth by the action of the teeth, tongue and the chewing muscles that pull the lower jaw upwards and move it sideways.

Three kinds of teeth make the process of mastication more efficient: sharp-edged cutters at the front (incisors), sharp-pointed tearers in the

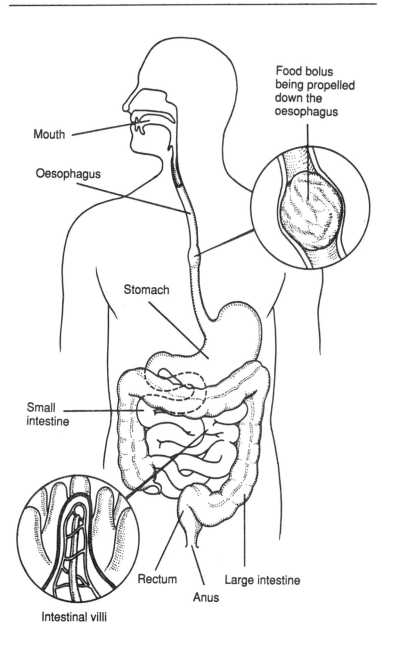

Mouth

Oesophagus

Food bolus being propelled down the oesophagus

Stomach

Small intestine

Rectum

Anus

Large intestine

Intestinal villi

Digestive system

middle (canines) and flat-topped grinders at the back (molars and premolars).

Chewing turns food into into a paste-like mass, which the tongue then pushes towards the back of the throat. Reflex swallowing propels this food bolus down the oesophagus into the stomach, a journey that takes only two to three seconds.

Mechanical breakdown of the food continues due to churning movements of the stomach walls. Acidic gastric juices released from glands in the stomach lining begin the breakdown of proteins within the food. After two to four hours in the stomach – sometimes longer when the consumption of alcohol has delayed the reflex emptying of the stomach – partially digested food, which is now in the form of a thick liquid, passes on gradually into the small intestine.

Through the duodenum, jejunum and ileum of the small intestine the digestive processes continue, to complete the breakdown of carbohydrates, fats and proteins into molecules small enough to be absorbed through the intestinal wall. To speed up the absorption of nutrient molecules, the inside lining of the small intestine is folded into millions of tiny projections, called villi, that massively increase the surface area in contact with the flow of digested food.

Movement of food along the small intestine is facilitated by peristalsis – continuous rhythmic contractions of the muscles in the intestinal wall. Digestion in the small intestine is aided by the action of bile, produced in the liver, stored in the gall bladder and released into the duodenum – as well as the chemical effects of several different enzymes secreted by the pancreas, also into the duodenum.

Bile assists in the digestion of fats; pancreatic enzymes break down proteins, fats and carbohydrates. The vitamins and minerals within food do not need to be digested before they can be absorbed. Within one to four hours, food will normally have reached the end of the small intestine, by which time all or most of the nutrients should have been absorbed.

Undigested matter leaving the small intestine then arrives in the last section of the gastrointestinal tract – the large intestine – which consists of the caecum, colon and rectum. Movement of the faeces (undigested matter) through the colon is again controlled by peristalsis. During the passage of faeces, most of its water and salt constituents are absorbed into the surrounding blood vessels.

The remainder of the faeces is then stored in the rectum as a semi-solid mass, ready to be expelled through the anus. Distension of the rectum by faeces is the stimulus that triggers the urge for a bowel movement.

Men appear to have a shorter transit time for the contents of their intestine than women, even when both sexes are eating the same amount of fibre in their diet. The transit time is known to vary from ten hours to as long as several days in some people, with a slower movement of faeces through the colon being associated with a greater risk of bowel cancer. This is one good reason to eat a diet high in fibre (*see* **Chapter 2**).

LIVER

The liver is the largest organ in the body and is situated in the upper right area of the abdominal cavity, mostly under the lower ribs on that side. It has many different functions, among them assisting with the processing of essential nutrients:

- bile produced by the liver helps with the digestion of fats in the small intestine
- cholesterol is formed in the liver from saturated fat in the diet – some cholesterol is used to form the membranes lining new cells and to make certain hormones; too much cholesterol is bad for your heart and circulation
- surplus glucose (sugar) is converted to glycogen (starch) in the liver and stored for future energy production
- surplus amino acids from digested protein can be converted by the liver into glucose or protein.

PANCREAS

The pancreas is a gland which lies across the back wall of the abdomen, just behind and under the stomach, with one end nestling in the curve made by the duodenum and the other end situated close to the spleen.

Digestive juices produced by the pancreas and released into the duodenum contain enzymes which help complete the chemical breakdown of fats, carbohydrates and proteins. They also contain an alkali, sodium bicarbonate, which neutralises the acids that enter the duodenum from the stomach.

Hormones released by the pancreas directly into the bloodstream include insulin and glucagon, which help control the absorption of sugar from the blood into cells throughout the body.

Kidneys and urinary system

The urinary system is designed to remove chemical waste and excess water from the body. In addition, the kidneys have a number of other important functions, including keeping the blood pressure under control.

The kidneys are a pair of bean-shaped organs surrounded by fat and situated on either side of the spine against the back wall of the abdominal cavity. Each is over 10cm long, 6cm wide and weighs nearly 0.5kg.

To fulfil its main function as an efficient filtration unit, each kidney contains around one million tiny filters known as nephrons. Each nephron starts off as a cup-shaped structure, Bowman's capsule, which surrounds a tuft of small blood vessels called the glomerulus.

Blood flowing into the glomerulus brings with it a wide range of cells and substances. Larger particles, such as red and white blood cells, platelets and blood proteins, are normally too big to filter through into the nephron. Substances consisting of smaller molecules, such as salts, glucose, minerals and chemical waste from the breakdown of worn-out cells, from muscle activity and from the processing of nutrients and drugs, are filtered from the blood into the tubule section of the nephron, along with large amounts of water.

The filtration that takes place in the glomerulus is only the first stage of the blood purification process. During its passage through the various tubule loops, the filtered liquid will lose most of its water content and controlled amounts of some of its dissolved substances back to the surrounding blood vessels. This is how the body regulates the salt and acid content of the bloodstream and keeps itself adequately hydrated.

To maintain a constant acidity level, a tight control is kept on how much acid and ammonia is taken back from the tubules. Over 80 litres of water filter through the kidneys every day, but about 99 per cent of this is returned from the tubules to the bloodstream. In hot weather,

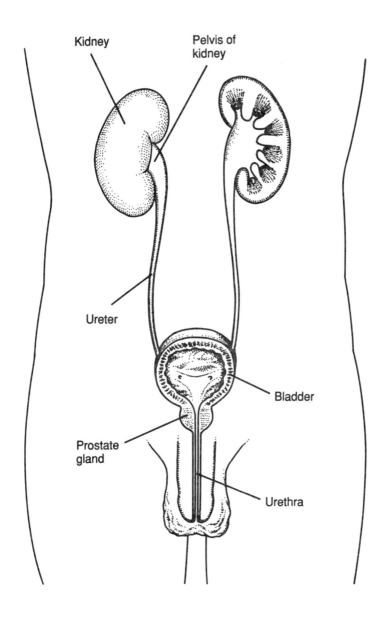

Kidneys and urinary system

when more fluid is being lost from the body in sweat, the amount of water re-absorbed from the tubules will be even greater. Therefore, unless this deficit is made up by drinking larger volumes, the urine produced by the kidneys will become more concentrated.

The waste fluid left behind in each nephron's tubule empties into a funnel-shaped cavity in the centre of the kidney – the renal pelvis – from where it drains into the ureter. Each kidney has its own ureter, a narrow muscular tube about 25–30cm long that carries urine to the bladder. Constant rhythmic contraction of the muscle in the ureter wall maintains a steady urine flow. Valves in the section of the ureter within the kidney, and the diagonal position of the ureter as it passes through the bladder wall, should prevent any backflow.

Lying behind the front section of the pelvic bone, in the mid-line, is the bladder, a muscular bag that acts as a temporary storage chamber for urine. The bladder is supported by powerful muscles in the floor of the pelvis. The urethra takes urine from the bladder along the length of the penis. A ring of muscle, known as a sphincter, surrounds the start of this narrow tube to prevent the release of urine until it is convenient.

OTHER KIDNEY FUNCTIONS

In addition to its blood filtration and purification function, the kidney:

- activates vitamin D, which helps maintain strong, healthy bones
- produces renin, a hormone which helps to control blood pressure
- releases erythropoietin, a hormone which stimulates red blood cell production by the bone marrow.

Passing urine

As the bladder fills up, the stretching of its muscle wall sends messages to the brain that are interpreted as the desire to pass urine. Typically, this desire will disappear for a time if it is ignored, only to keep recurring at increasingly shorter intervals, until it is present constantly and too intense to ignore any longer.

When you have been drinking alcohol, you are likely to miss out the gentle early-warning signs, explaining why a visit to the toilet may suddenly become an urgent need. This is because alcohol may reduce your sensitivity to bladder impulses. It also increases the volume of urine being produced, causing the bladder to fill up more rapidly.

To urinate, the sphincter muscle around the entrance to the urethra is relaxed and as the bladder empties its muscle wall contracts to push out the urine. If the bladder is not emptied voluntarily, it will eventually empty itself spontaneously.

Endocrine system

The endocrine system consists of a collection of glands which release a variety of chemicals known as hormones into the bloodstream. Although these hormones circulate throughout the whole body, each one targets specific tissues or organs which are programmed to respond to it.

Many different aspects of physical and mental function are activated and controlled by hormones, including growth, sexual development, response to stress and cell metabolism (energy-producing and -consuming processes). The greater the concentration of a particular hormone which is circulating in the blood, the stronger its effects will be, assuming the target tissues and organs are responding normally.

To understand how the endocrine system works, it is easiest to consider each component in turn, starting with the two control centres in the brain. The hypothalamus, situated on the underside of the brain, exerts overall control of the endocrine system. Activity in the pituitary gland (*see below*) is influenced by both nerve impulses and by a selection of hormones released from the hypothalamus. Psychological stimuli, such as fear, anger or sexual arousal, are able to trigger physical changes in the body by altering activity in the hypothalamus, which in turn influences the production and release of different hormones by the pituitary and other glands.

The pituitary gland, also located at the base of the brain and connected to the hypothalamus by a short stalk, produces a variety of its own hormones, as well as controlling hormone production by other endocrine glands. Pituitary hormones include:

- growth hormone, which regulates body growth and development
- antidiuretic hormone, which increases water reabsorption from the kidney tubules

- thyroid stimulating hormone (TSH), which maintains consistent production of thyroid hormones by the thyroid gland
- adrenocorticotrophic hormone (ACTH), which maintains consistent production of cortisol by the adrenal glands.

Thyroid gland

Hormones produced by the thyroid gland stimulate metabolism in nearly every cell in the body and help maintain body temperature. Situated at the front of the neck, the thyroid gland also assists the control of calcium levels in the blood through the action of an additional hormone called calcitonin.

The small parathyroid glands, situated within the thyroid gland, produce parathyroid hormone, which has the opposite effect to calcitonin on blood calcium levels. If the concentration of calcium in the blood is too low, an increased output of parathyroid hormone restores the calcium level to normal.

Pancreas

In addition to its production of digestive enzymes (*see page 18*), the pancreas releases two hormones into the bloodstream – insulin and glucagon – which together control the concentration of glucose (sugar) in the blood.

Adrenal glands

This pair of small, triangular glands fits like a cap on top of each kidney. Hormones produced by the adrenal glands include:

- aldosterone, which is released in response to the action of renin from the kidney to control the body's salt and water balance
- cortisol (hydrocortisone), which is released in response to the action of ACTH from the pituitary gland to control the body's use of carbohydrates, fats and proteins; it also suppresses excessive inflammatory reactions and assists recovery from injury, illness or surgery
- adrenaline, which is released in response to nerve stimulation from the hypothalamus as a reaction to stress, fear or excitement. The actions of adrenaline are the basis of the primitive 'fight or flight' response (*see pages 19–20*) and include a faster rate of breathing and more rapid pulse

- androgens, which are continuously released in small amounts from the adrenal glands and, along with androgens produced by the testicles, are important in the development and maintenance of strong healthy bones and muscles.

Testicles

Specialised cells in the testicles produce several androgen hormones, the most potent of which is testosterone, in response to the release of gonadotrophin hormones from the pituitary gland. Androgens from the testicles are more active than adrenal gland androgens; they stimulate the appearance of male sexual characteristics at puberty, including enlargement of the penis, growth of facial and body hair, and increased bulk of the muscles, particularly around the chest and shoulders. Testicular androgens, like the adrenal androgens, also stimulate bone and muscle growth.

Brain and nervous system

The brain is the control centre of the body. At all times, even during sleep, the brain receives, sorts, interprets and stores information transmitted as nerve impulses from every part of the body.

Some of this sensory information results in conscious awareness of an outside event or internal change in the body. The brain may then initiate a controlled movement in response to this sensation. However, a lot of the incoming data simply triggers an automatic or reflex adjustment, such as a change in posture or alteration in blood flow, of which the individual is not aware.

The brain is also the seat of emotion, instinct and intellect. It is the memory store which records experiences and enables the individual to learn. The brain determines personality, behaviour, creativity and talent for physical and mental tasks.

Brain structure

Weighing over 1kg and containing over 100 billion nerve cells, the brain occupies most of the space inside the skull. In addition to the skull's bony protection, a layer of cerebrospinal fluid (CSF) between two of the three outer brain membranes (meninges) provides extra cushioning to reduce the risk of damage to the sensitive nerve cells.

The largest section of the brain is the cerebrum, which is divided into two almost identical hemispheres connected by a large bundle of nerve fibres called the corpus callosum. The thin outer surface of these hemispheres – the cerebral cortex – is folded into a number of different lobes, separated by deep clefts and named after the skull bones that lie directly over them: frontal, temporal, parietal and occipital lobes.

Only a few areas of the cerebral cortex are known to have specific functions, such as initiating movement, responding to visual images, or understanding language.

Beneath the six layers of nerve cells that make up the cerebral cortex (the so-called grey matter), much of the remainder of the cerebrum consists of nerve tracts (the white matter), which connect various areas of the cortex together. These tracts are also linked to a number of important nerve centres deeper within the brain, including:

- the hypothalamus, which helps control appetite, thirst and body temperature and influences sleep, aggression and sexual behaviour
- the pituitary gland, which produces a variety of hormones and controls other endocrine glands (*see page 23*)
- the limbic system, which handles emotions, processes smell sensations and is involved in registration and recall of memories
- the basal ganglia, which control complex body movements through connections to the cerebellum
- the cerebellum, which is concerned with balance, muscle co-ordination and posture.

Brain stem and spinal cord

Just in front of the cerebellum, passing downwards from the middle of the underside of the cerebrum, is a thick stalk which carries major nerve tracts running between the brain and spinal cord, and *vice versa*. Inside this brain stem are the nerve centres which control heartbeat and breathing.

Below the brain stem, the spinal cord runs down through a large hole in the base of the skull and passes on down a canal in the centre of the spinal column. The brain and spinal cord together form the central nervous system (CNS). Nerves from the peripheral nervous system run into and out of the spinal cord between adjacent pairs of vertebrae.

Peripheral nervous system

This part of the nervous system consists of sensory nerves, which carry information from all areas of the body to the CNS, along with motor nerves, which take instructions from the CNS out to individual groups of muscles to initiate movement.

Nerve impulses arriving from sensory nerve fibres may be carried up the spinal cord and brain stem into the part of the cerebral cortex designed to analyse and interpret them. The brain may then initiate a response which passes as nerve impulses down through the brain stem and spinal cord, emerging along specific motor nerve fibres to cause a particular muscle to contract.

Because the nerve tracts cross, movement of the right-hand side of the body is controlled by the left side of the brain, and the left-hand side by the right side of the brain.

Muscles normally controlled by the brain may respond as an automatic reflex, for example, in reaction to a painful stimulus. In this situation, the sensory signal that reaches the spinal cord makes direct contact with the motor nerve nearby, without having to pass up to the brain first. Reflexes are important as a protective mechanism: for example, they make it possible for you to pull your hand quickly away from something that is hot enough to cause a burn.

The brain, however, can override a reflex, for example, allowing you to walk across burning ashes, or consciously suppressing contraction of the muscles on the front of the thigh when a doctor tests the knee-jerk reflex.

Autonomic nervous system

This part of the nervous system is concerned with body functions that work without conscious control. Autonomic nerves regulate blood pressure, sweating, skin blood flow, sexual arousal, including erection and ejaculation, body temperature and the passage of intestinal contents by peristalsis.

The autonomic nervous system is divided into sympathetic nerves, which trigger the 'fight or flight' response to dangerous or frightening situations, and parasympathetic nerves which are primarily involved in body functions at rest or asleep.

Most of the autonomic nerve cells run parallel to the spine as a chain of linked clumps known as ganglia, with autonomic fibres passing along the same routes as some of the nerves from the peripheral nervous system.

Eyes

The eye is a fluid-filled ball, roughly spherical in shape, that is held inside a bony socket in the skull by three pairs of muscles, which also control its movement.

Most of the focusing in the eye is done by the cornea, the front part of the tough outer coating of the eye, which is transparent and shaped like a dome. Light passes through the cornea and then on through a hole in the centre of the iris, known as the pupil.

Additional focusing is done by the lens in each eye. This elastic, transparent structure is suspended within a circular ring of muscle, known as the ciliary body. Contraction or relaxation of this muscle changes the shape of the lens, allowing the eye to focus on a particular object by accurately directing all the light rays to cross each other on the surface of the retina at the back of the eye.

The amount of light entering the eye is controlled by the action of muscle fibres within the iris. In dark conditions, radial fibres contract as a reflex to widen the pupil and let more light in. When there is bright light, circular fibres contract to narrow the pupil.

Visualising an image

Millions of light-sensitive cells in the retina – rods and cones – convert these light signals into nerve impulses, which are then transferred to the brain along the optic nerve. Rods are concerned with the fine detail of an image, cones are each sensitive to one of the three primary colours: red, blue or yellow.

The image formed on the retina is actually upside down, but as part of its ability to interpret the nerve impulses it receives from each eye, the brain learns to turn the picture the correct way up. Images are assembled in the visual cortex at the back of the brain.

Crossover of some of the optic nerve fibres behind the eyes means that both sides of the brain receive signals from both eyes. Because the images from the two eyes differ slightly, the brain is able to produce a three-dimensional view of its surroundings, judging depth as well as height and width. Two eyes also offer a wider field of vision.

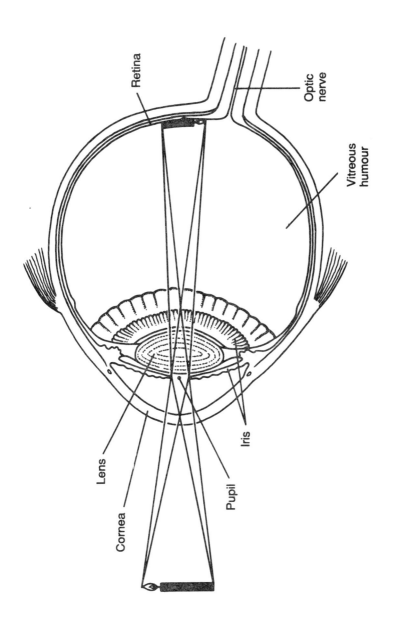

Eye structure

EYE PROTECTION

The eyelids close quickly as a reflex mechanism when any object approaches the eye. A row of tiny glands on each eyelid produces small amounts of an oil that stops the lids sticking together when the eyes are closed, as well as contributing to the thin sheet of tears that constantly bathes the eye. Eyelashes are strong, curved hairs arranged in two rows along the front edge of each eyelid. They trap particles of dust and grit blown into the eye.

Tears are produced by glands inside the upper and outer margins of the bony eye socket and also by glands in the conjunctiva, a thin layer of transparent skin over the front of the eye and under the eyelids. Blinking sweeps a film of tears across the eye, keeping its surface well lubricated and washing away dust and dirt. In addition to salty water, tears contain a natural antiseptic.

Tears drain through a single hole near the inner end of each eyelid, first into small tear sacs and then into the nose, which is why your nose may run when you cry.

Ears and hearing

The ear is designed to pick up sound waves – rhythmic, rapid pressure changes in the surrounding air produced by vibrating objects – and to convert these sound waves into electrical signals that can be interpreted by the brain. There are three main sections to each ear.

Outer ear

The visible part of the ear, known as the pinna, consists of a cartilage skeleton covered with skin. Although it helps funnel sound waves towards the eardrum, you would still be able to hear without it.

Sound then passes along a skin-lined passage – the auditory canal – which is about 2cm long, before striking the eardrum and causing it to vibrate. Wax is produced by glands within the lining of this canal, normally in small amounts that clear naturally. Along with the hairs at the entrance to the ear, the wax traps dirt and dust particles.

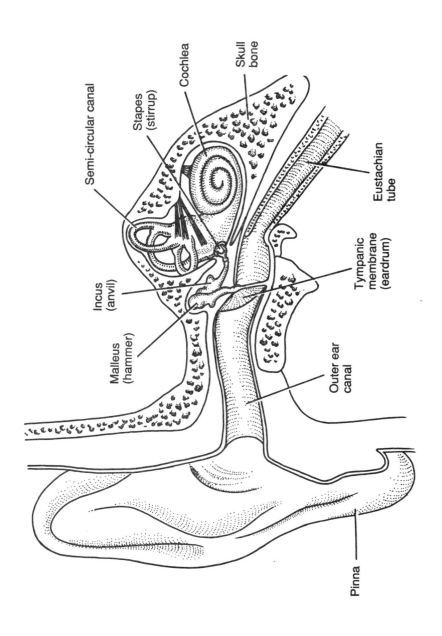

Ear structure

The eardrum is a delicate membrane that separates the outer and middle ear; when healthy it vibrates in sympathy with the incoming sound waves.

Middle ear
This small air-filled cavity is crossed by three tiny, moveable and inter-linked bones (the hammer, anvil and stirrup). Vibrations of the eardrum are amplified as they are transmitted across these bones to a window in the outside wall of the inner ear.

To keep the air pressure inside the middle ear equal to the air pressure against the outside of the eardrum, and thereby allow the eardrum to vibrate freely, the middle ear cavity is connected to the back of the throat by the eustachian tube.

Inner ear
The hearing part of the inner ear, the cochlea, consists of a spiral membrane, known as the basilar membrane, bathed in fluid that starts to vibrate in response to incoming vibrations from the middle ear. The spiral structure of the cochlea resembles a small snail shell.

Different sections of the membrane vibrate according to the exact frequency of the pressure waves. Hair cells lining the vibrating part of the membrane are also set in motion and because each of these hairs is connected to a nerve fibre the vibration is converted into an electrical impulse.

A pattern of electrical impulses, corresponding to the incoming pattern of sound waves, is then conveyed to the brain along the auditory nerve. In the part of the brain where these signals are processed – the auditory cortex – they are interpreted as a particular sound on the basis of previous experiences of sound held in the memory.

Finally, at the back of the inner ear, three fluid-filled semi-circular canals at right angles to each other help to maintain balance by detecting even the slightest body movement.

Smell, taste and touch
Smell

Microscopic chemical particles carried in the air are detected as a particular smell by sensitive hair-like nerve endings lining the roof of the nose. These odorous molecules become trapped in the secretions produced by the mucous lining of the nose and when they come into contact with the olfactory nerve filaments, electrical impulses are relayed to the base of the brain. Different types of particle relating to different odours stimulate their own unique pattern of nerve impulses, which can then be interpreted by the brain on the basis of previous experience.

Taste

About 10,000 taste buds are positioned on the top and sides of the tongue, as well as being scattered over the roof and back of the mouth. There are four main taste sensations: sweetness, detected by taste buds at the tip of the tongue; bitterness, by those at the back of the tongue; sourness, by those in the middle of the tongue sides; and saltiness by taste buds at the front of the tongue sides.

Chemicals in food or drink dissolve in saliva and then penetrate pores in the tongue surface to reach the underlying taste buds. Stimulation of a taste bud triggers an electrical impulse in the attached nerve fibre, which is transmitted to the brain for interpretation.

Although the taste buds can only distinguish the four basic tastes, a wide range of flavours can be appreciated through the involvement of smell receptors in the nose. These are stimulated by food odours passing up from the back of the throat, which is why anyone with a nose blocked by mucus due to a cold is likely to experience a marked loss of taste.

Touch

Buried in the skin are many types of sensory receptors which respond to different forms of external stimulation, such as fine touch, pressure, pain, heat and cold. Some of these receptors are just a single nerve fibre wrapped around an individual hair so that it can respond to any movement of that hair. Others are more complex, containing several layers of cells, with nerve fibres arranged in a loop or coil.

Signals are carried from these receptors along sensory nerves to the spinal cord (*see page 26*) and on up to the area of the brain, known as the sensory cortex, where different skin sensations are processed and interpreted.

Some areas of skin are more sensitive to painful stimuli, or better able to discriminate between close points of touch, because they contain a greater number of the appropriate receptors. Also, the most sensitive parts of the body, including the hands, feet, lips and genitals, are represented by larger areas of the sensory cortex.

Skin, hair and nails

Skin

The skin does a lot more than just hold the organs and fluids of the body together. This complex structure, which itself is one of the body's largest organs, weighing over 4kg and covering a total area of over 2 square metres, performs the following different functions:

- stops body tissue absorbing water like a sponge, while retaining enough moisture to stay supple
- keeps out bacteria and chemicals
- uses the sun's ultraviolet rays to manufacture vitamin D
- responds to pain, touch, temperature and pressure, sending this information to the brain for processing and interpretation
- controls body temperature.

Epidermal layer

The epidermis is the thin outer layer of skin. On its surface, there are layers of flat dead cells which contain a type of protein known as keratin. This is what provides the skin with its tough, waterproof protective coating.

The dead skin cells are continuously being discarded, particularly when you wash or dry your body. Areas of the body that experience the most wear and tear, such as the palms and soles, develop a thicker layer of these protective cells.

To replace the outer skin cells, new, living epidermal cells are continuously produced underneath them. It normally takes about four weeks for the new cells to migrate to the skin surface, dying on the way up.

Special skin cells called melanocytes produce the pigment melanin that helps shield the body from the sun's ultraviolet rays and gives the skin its colour. The degree of pigmentation depends on the number and activity of these melanocytes, which is primarily genetically determined. Melanin production can be stimulated by regular sun exposure to produce a tan.

Dermal layer

Much thicker than the epidermis, the dermis contains connective tissues which give the skin both resilience and elasticity. Embedded within this connective tissue are a variety of specialised structures, including sweat and sebaceous (oil-producing) glands, sensory receptors and hair follicles. There is also a network of tiny blood vessels to keep the cells supplied with oxygen and nutrients.

Subcutaneous layer

Below the dermis is a layer of subcutaneous fat, which varies in thickness around the body. These fat cells can act as a source of reserve fuel and also provide protection and insulation for internal body organs.

Hair function and growth

Hair is basically composed of dead cells plus keratin, the protein also found in skin. Each shaft of hair consists of a spongy semi-hollow core (the medulla), made of soft rectangular cells; a surrounding layer of long, thin fibres (the cortex), made of cells which become harder as they emerge from the scalp or skin; and an outer layer of overlapping, flat cells (the cuticle) arranged like slates on a roof.

The root of each hair is firmly enclosed by a cluster of living cells at the base of the hair follicle, known as the bulb, which produce keratin while the hair is actively growing. Within the bulb is a mass of cells – the papilla – and nerve endings, which explains why pulling out a hair is painful.

Each hair grows for a period lasting between two and five years, before entering the so-called resting phase. As growth stops, the bulb pulls back from the hair root and the hair falls out. After about three months, a new hair begins to grow, to take its place.

Different hairs enter this resting phase at different times, resulting in a variable loss of scalp hair of anything between 50 and 150 hairs each day.

The pigment melanin gives hair its colour. Red or auburn hair results from varying amounts of the red type of melanin; colours ranging from black to blonde depend on the proportion of the brown type of melanin. Hair turns white or grey when the production of melanin ceases.

Nails

Not only do nails protect the tips of the fingers and toes, they also assist the manipulation of an object and provide a useful tool for scratching.

Each nail consists of a hard curved plate made of keratin, the same protein that is found in skin and hair. The base of the nail plate is paler than the rest of it and shaped like a half moon; overlying this area of nail is a flap of free skin known as the cuticle.

Under the nail plate, at the base of the nail bed, is the area of tissue from which the nail grows. Fingernails normally grow at a rate of about 1cm every three months, so it takes up to five months to grow a completely new nail on the finger. Toenails grow at least twice as slowly, which is why you don't have to cut them so often.

Bones and joints

Bone consists of a tough, rubbery protein called collagen, which is impregnated with the minerals calcium and phosphorus to make it rigid. The resultant structure is light, but incredibly strong.

An outer, hard layer, known as cortical bone, surrounds a spongy core which contains the liquid bone marrow. While the shafts of the long bones are mainly hollow, the ends are filled with this spongy type of bone, arranged in struts to provide added strength.

A dense membrane, the periosteum, lines the outside of all bones. Blood vessels running in the periosteum and through canals in the cortical bone keep the bone tissue alive by supplying nutrients and oxygen. They also take away the new blood cells being continuously produced by the bone marrow (*see page 41*).

A total of 206 bones usually makes up the framework of an adult skeleton, although some people have an extra pair of ribs, or an additional bone in their hands or feet. There are no major differences between the skeleton of a man and a woman. However, bones are usually larger and heavier in men and the pelvis narrower.

In addition to providing a supporting structure and anchorage for the skeletal muscles, bone has several other important functions:

- protection of delicate internal organs, such as the brain and heart
- blood cell production in bone marrow, mainly within flat bones such as the pelvis, ribs, sternum and skull
- supply of calcium into the bloodstream when required.

Bone growth and healing

As a child grows, new bone is formed from cartilage plates that lie across the shaft, near each end of the long bones. Cartilage is changed into bone on the side of this epiphyseal plate nearest the centre of the bone, but the thickness of the plate remains the same as new cartilage is formed on its outer surface. These changes are stimulated by the action of growth hormone, causing the bones to lengthen.

Growth ceases in early adult life when the epiphyseal plates are entirely converted into bone. However, the two types of bone cell which are involved in the formation of new bone – osteoblasts and osteoclasts – continue to function within the bones, to keep their internal structure strong and healthy.

After a fracture, the osteoblasts and osteoclasts assist the repair process. Osteoblasts lay down new collagen within the blood clot that forms between the broken ends. Osteoclasts remove unwanted bone debris and release minerals which can be re-used in the formation of new bone.

Bone tissues are alive: new bone forms and old bone degenerates throughout life. This activity slows down with advancing years, which explains why older men have weaker bones that are more likely to fracture.

Various hormones control bone metabolism in men, including testosterone, adrenal hormones, parathyroid hormone and growth hormone. As there is no major change in one of the controlling hormones, men are less vulnerable to osteoporosis than women, who at the menopause gradually lose the beneficial action of the female sex hormone oestrogen on their bones.

Joint structure and movement

Joints are the junctions where bones meet. Not all joints move – there are fixed joints in the skull which fuse in childhood once the head has stopped growing.

In a mobile joint, the ends where the bones meet have a protective covering of cartilage, which provides a smooth, low-friction but hard-wearing surface. A fibrous capsule surrounds and protects the joint, and inside this capsule some joints have a thin synovial membrane which releases small amounts of fluid. This synovial fluid acts as a joint

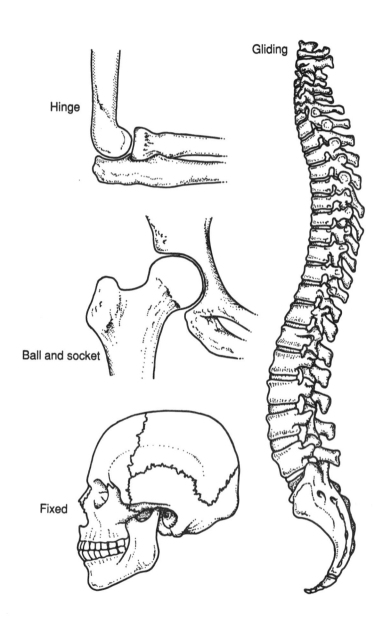

Examples of joints in the body

lubricant, as well as keeping the internal cartilage surfaces supplied with oxygen and nutrients.

A joint moves as a result of either the contraction of muscles that pass across it, or the pull of a tendon on one of the bones. Although the amount of movement in each different direction is determined primarily by the shape of the internal joint surfaces, tough bands of elastic tissue called ligaments normally prevent overstretching of a joint.

The main types of joint, each with their own characteristic range of movements, are:

- ball and socket joints, which allow movement of one bone in all directions; e.g. shoulder, hip
- hinge joints, which move in one plane only; e.g. elbow (the knee is not just a hinge joint, as it also allows the lower leg to rotate)
- pivot joints, which allow rotation only; e.g. joint between upper two neck bones
- gliding joints, which allow movement between two almost flat or slightly curved surfaces; e.g. spinal joints
- ellipsoidal joints, which consist of an oval protrusion fitting into an oval hollow, allowing all movements except rotation; e.g. wrist joint
- saddle joints, where the surfaces curve outward in one direction and inward in the other; e.g. the joint at the base of the thumb
- fixed joints, skull suture joints allow no movement in adults; sacroiliac joints on either side of the back of the pelvis permit only slight movement.

Skeletal muscles

Skeletal muscles are attached to the bones, either directly or via tendons formed from the outer muscle sheath. They maintain body posture and generate movements of the head, trunk and limbs.

Skeletal muscles are under conscious control (see peripheral nervous system, *page 27*). Stimulation of a muscle by its incoming motor nerve causes the fibres within it to contract. This contraction involves the sliding movement of specialised proteins, arranged as parallel overlapping rods inside the hundreds of long filaments that make up each muscle fibre. The muscle fibres are shortened in proportion to the amount of overlap.

To move a particular part of the body, usually one group of skeletal muscles is contracted while the group with the opposite action is relaxed. Muscles are broadly classified according to the type of movement they perform: for example, adductors move part of the body inwards, abductors move it outwards, levators raise it and depressors lower it. Extensor muscles open a joint, flexors close it.

Cardiac and smooth muscle

These other two types of muscle in the body are controlled unconsciously by the autonomic nervous system (*see page 27*). Contraction and relaxation of these muscles change the shape or volume of internal structures, such as organs and blood vessels.

Cardiac muscle (the myocardium), which makes up the walls of the four heart chambers, is designed to continuously pump blood out into the circulation. Smooth muscle is arranged in circular bands around blood vessels to control their diameter and thus the flow of blood. The intestine has smooth muscle fibres around its circumference as well as along the length of the wall. Regular contraction and relaxation of these muscle bands produces a movement known as peristalsis, which squeezes the intestinal contents forwards.

Blood and lymph

In an adult man, about six litres of blood flow through the circulation system. Just over half of this volume is a pale, amber substance known as plasma, 90 per cent of which is water in which a wide variety of constituents are dissolved, including various salts, nutrients, enzymes, antibodies and blood-clotting proteins. The remaining 45 or so per cent of the blood volume is made up of red blood cells, platelets and white blood cells. The purpose of blood is:

- to carry oxygen and nutrients to every cell in the body
- to remove carbon dioxide and other waste products from tissues (for elimination through the lungs and kidneys)
- to seal up any damage to a blood vessel, through the formation of a blood clot
- to provide a highly mobile defence system against invading organisms.

Red blood cells

These flat, disc-shaped cells are constantly being made in the bone marrow, from where they are fed into the bloodstream. They carry oxygen into the tissues, where they exchange it for carbon dioxide which they then return to the lungs. Haemoglobin, a pigment made from iron, is the component of the red blood cell designed to gather and release oxygen. There are about five million red blood cells per cubic millimetre of blood.

Platelets

These round, flattened particles, also produced in the bone marrow, are the smallest type of blood cell in the circulation. There are about 250,000 platelets per cubic millimetre of blood.

Platelets play a key role in the process of blood clotting. In contact with a damaged vessel wall, the platelets become chemically activated and, as a result, start to clump together to plug the hole. Activated platelets also release chemicals that stimulate the formation of fibrin from other blood-clotting substances which are being carried in the plasma.

Filaments of fibrin combine with clumps of platelets and also with red and white blood cells to form a solid blood clot. The sealing of damaged blood vessels with a clot helps to keep the amount of blood lost from the circulation to a minimum.

White blood cells

Several different types of white blood cell are found in the circulation, together totalling about 7,500 per cubic millimetre of blood. White blood cells are also made in the bone marrow, but they mature in several other tissues in the body, including the lymph nodes, the spleen, tonsils and the thymus, which is a gland situated behind the breast bone.

The lifespan of a white blood cell is highly variable. Some may last for many years, others for only a few hours. During an infection, millions of white cells may be destroyed while dealing with the invading bugs.

Unlike red blood cells, which are confined to the bloodstream, white blood cells are able to push their way through the walls of both blood and lymph vessels (see lymphatic system below), thereby reaching the site of an infection, tumour or injury.

Varieties of white blood cell include:

- neutrophils, which directly attack and engulf invading bugs, often with the formation of pus consisting of dead neutrophils and bacteria
- basophils, which release chemicals that trigger allergic and inflammatory reactions
- eosinophils, which proliferate in response to allergic reactions or parasite infections
- monocytes, which can enlarge to become macrophages that penetrate infected tissue and, like neutrophils, engulf and kill bacteria and other organisms
- lymphocytes, which can target, neutralise and destroy foreign cells, including micro-organisms, tumour cells and substances that provoke an allergic reaction.

BLOOD GROUPS

Red blood cells in the circulation carry certain types of protein on their surface called antigens. Everyone's blood can be classified into a particular blood group, based on the presence or absence of antigens.
. The main antigens are those from the ABO system, along with the rhesus antigen, to produce four basic blood groups: AB, A, B and O, all either rhesus positive or rhesus negative. Before a blood transfusion, the doctor will check that the donated blood is compatible with the patient's blood group to avoid an unpleasant, potentially fatal, reaction.

Lymphatic system

The thin-walled transparent vessels that make up the lymphatic system start as blind-ended capillaries, which penetrate most body tissues. These lymph capillaries drain into larger lymphatic vessels, which have internal valves to ensure there is no backflow.

Lymph, a clear, protein-rich fluid, passes towards the heart through this network of vessels, driven by pressure from the contraction of surrounding muscles together with the constant pressure changes inside the abdominal and chest cavities. The majority of lymph vessels run alongside the arteries and veins of the blood circulation.

Scattered throughout the body are bean-shaped lymph nodes, each of which receives lymph from one or more lymphatic vessels and drains it into at least one exit vessel. These lymph nodes are located under the arms, in the groins and around the neck, as well as deep in the chest and abdomen. There is also a similar type of lymph tissue, situated in the liver and spleen.

Having passed through these lymph nodes, lymph drains through to the upper part of the chest, emptying ultimately into the bloodstream through the large veins at the base of the neck.

The three main functions of the lymphatic system are:

- to absorb digested fats from the small intestine
- to collect up protein and water that the blood circulation has left behind in the tissues
- to assist the body's immune system (*see below*).

Immune system

To protect the body from the millions of harmful bugs, chemicals and other substances that bombard it over a lifetime, there is a complex network of natural defences known as the immune system. The main task of the immune system is to neutralise and destroy micro-organisms, such as bacteria or viruses, which could otherwise seriously damage body organs or tissues, either by infecting them or by releasing toxins that poison their cells.

The first line of defence consists of various physical and chemical barriers to infection, which together are classified as the body's innate immune system. These different barriers include:

- antimicrobial substances present in saliva, tears and sweat
- acids in the stomach, which kill most micro-organisms
- friendly bacteria in the intestine and on the skin, which restrict the growth of harmful micro-organisms
- mucus in the nose and other airways, which traps micro-organisms and is then either swallowed, sneezed or coughed up.

Any micro-organism or foreign substance that bypasses the innate immune system is immediately attacked by white blood cells – the adaptive immune system. These cells can destroy invaders by means of several different mechanisms:

- some lymphocytes produce antibodies, which latch on to one of the surface proteins (antigens) of the invaders, either killing them, or making it easier for other white blood cells to devour them
- other lymphocytes, which are able to target the invader directly, may multiply rapidly and then attack the invading micro-organisms or the offending tumour cells
- certain white blood cells, like eosinophils and basophils, deal with a foreign cell or substance by releasing chemicals that assist the function of the lymphocytes and macrophages.

In addition to circulating in the bloodstream, lymphocytes congregate in the lymph nodes ready to deal with micro-organisms that have been drawn into the lymphatic system from surrounding tissues. In this way an infection may be kept localised, instead of spreading to the rest of the body, which is why, for example, an infected finger may cause tender, swollen lymph nodes under the arm. Lymph tissue in the liver and spleen is designed to filter out and destroy micro-organisms being carried in the bloodstream.

Immunity

Immunity is the ability to recognise an invading micro-organism previously encountered, allowing the immune system to respond rapidly to any subsequent attack before the infection has time to take hold. This phenomenon is the result of the formation of a 'memory' cell from one type of lymphocyte, which carries an exact blueprint of the invader's distinguishing antigen.

Immunisation is the exposure of the body to a weakened or dead strain of a particular type of micro-organism, which artificially stimulates immunity to that infection (*see pages 88–9*).

Male reproductive system

The male reproductive system has three main functions: the production and storage of sperm; the production and release of sperm-containing seminal fluid during ejaculation; and the production of the male sex hormone testosterone.

While most men are aware of the basic anatomy of their genitals, certainly of the visible parts, there is a great deal of ignorance about what goes on beneath the surface. Understanding the position and

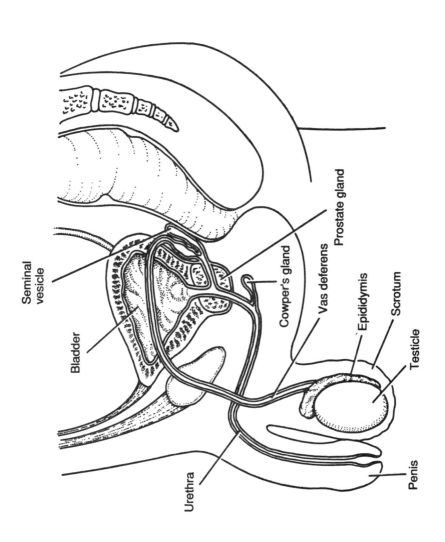

Male reproductive system

function of structures like the prostate gland and the vas deferens will be useful, for example, if you ever have problems with an enlarged prostate, or you are going to have a vasectomy (*see pages 129–32*).

Penis

Inside the penis are three cylinders of spongy tissue, two on the upper side, known as the corpora cavernosa, and one on the underside, the corpus spongiosum. When the penis is flaccid these three chambers are squashed flat; sexual stimulation causes the corpora cavernosa to become engorged with blood through a network of blood vessels, resulting in an erection.

Down through the corpus spongiosum runs the urethra, which is a muscular tube about 25cm long that carries urine and semen to the tip of the penis. The glans, the head of the penis, which is the end of the corpus spongiosum, is covered in uncircumcised men by a loose fold of skin called the prepuce or foreskin.

Testicles

These two sex glands, the male equivalent of the female's ovaries, manufacture sperm and the sex hormone testosterone. They hang together, but at different heights, within a wrinkled pouch of skin known as the scrotum, which is located below and behind the penis.

There is a good reason for positioning the testicles within the scrotum rather than inside the abdomen. The circulation of air around the scrotum keeps the testicles at a temperature around 5°C lower than the normal body temperature. This appears to enhance both sperm production and the release of testosterone.

Within each testicle are about 1,000 tiny tubes, coiled up like spaghetti. Unravelled and laid end to end, these would span a length of nearly 500 metres. Cells inside these seminiferous tubules start to produce immature sperm from puberty onwards, with each sperm taking about ten weeks to become fully developed. All the seminiferous tubules feed into the epididymis, which is a tightly coiled tube lying behind the testicle. In the epididymis, the sperm are stored and continue to mature over two to three weeks, after which they are ready to be ejaculated. As many as 500 million mature sperm reach the end of the epididymis each day.

A mature sperm cell is only about 0.05mm long and consists of a head, neck, midpiece, tail and endpiece. Healthy sperm have an oval-shaped head, which contains the genetic material that the father will contribute to his child should conception take place. The rest of the sperm is designed solely to generate the whip-like movements of the tail that propel it along.

Testosterone, a natural anabolic steroid hormone, is produced by specialised cells, known as Leydig cells, scattered between the lines of seminiferous tubules within each testicle. The production of testosterone by the testicles increases at puberty to cause the characteristic physical changes (*see page 53*).

Vas deferens

Prior to ejaculation, sperm are transported from the epididymis through a long duct, the vas deferens, towards the entrance to the urethra. About 60 per cent of the seminal fluid produced during ejaculation is released by the seminal vesicles into the vas deferens, to join the sperm on the way to the urethra.

Prostate

The prostate gland, which is normally the size of a chestnut in the adult male, is situated at the base of the bladder and surrounds the urethra. Secretions produced by the prostate are added to the seminal fluid while it is collecting at the start of the urethra, a few seconds before ejaculation occurs.

SEMEN

This thick, milky fluid, produced by the seminal vesicles and prostate gland, is added to sperm before ejaculation to provide nourishment for the millions of sperm cells. In the average man, the volume of semen released in one ejaculation is one teaspoonful or less.

Although about 90 per cent of semen is water, it contains a variety of essential nutrients, including zinc, potassium, glucose and vitamin C, which keep the ejaculated sperm alive and kicking.

Sexual arousal and responses

A wide variety of stimuli can sexually excite a man, causing a burst of electrical impulses from nerve centres close to the spinal cord, which produces an erection. This reflex response is controlled by other nerve centres in the brain, which react positively to erotic sensations. It may also be suppressed by feelings such as anxiety and guilt leading to loss of erection or failure to get an erection in the first place.

Different men respond to different erotic stimuli. Men are said to be more responsive to visual eroticism than women, but it is always dangerous to make these sorts of generalisations. A vital part of any sexual relationship is discovering what turns you on and letting your partner know how to get you aroused – and *vice versa*, of course.

Erections may also occur spontaneously during the dreaming phases of sleep and men commonly wake with an erection in the morning, although, more often than not, there will be no recollection of an erotic dream.

Two American experts in human sexuality, Masters and Johnson, were the first to produce (in 1966) a detailed description of the various phases of sexual response in men.

Excitation phase   The first stage of sexual arousal, the development of an erection, is the result of engorgement of the penis with blood, causing its spongy tissues to increase in length and volume and the overlying skin to stretch taut. An erection may come on within a few seconds or build up gradually, depending on the individual and the intensity of arousal. Muscles at the base of the penis are also stimulated to contract, maintaining the erection by preventing blood from escaping.

Plateau phase   The name of this, the second stage of sexual arousal, is misleading because it is one of progressive increase in sexual tension. In addition to the penis becoming erect, the lower part of the glans swells and the testicles enlarge to one-and-a-half times their resting size as a result of becoming engorged with blood. The testicles are also pulled upwards closer to the body.

The man's skin may start to flush red and usually his pulse, blood pressure and breathing rate will increase, owing to nerve activation rather than exertion. A few drops of clear, sticky fluid may seep out of the urethra at the tip of the penis, to lubricate the foreskin and neutralise any traces of urine that might otherwise harm the sperm about to be ejaculated. Because these secretions (which come from the Cowper's glands under the prostate) may occasionally contain sperm,

UNDERSTANDING THE MALE BODY

there is a risk that pregnancy may result from unprotected intercourse with a woman even without ejaculation.

Emission phase   If sexual stimulation continues for long enough during the plateau phase, preparation for ejaculation begins with an emission phase that lasts just a few seconds and from which there is no turning back. Contraction of the seminal vesicles massages semen into the vas deferens to join the sperm moving towards the start of the urethra. As sperm and semen arrive in the urethra, it stretches to accommodate this fluid and contraction of the prostate gland adds further seminal secretions.

Muscles at the entrance to the urethra from the bladder are normally tightly contracted at this stage to prevent semen escaping backwards, and urine from being passed out during ejaculation.

Orgasm phase   The muscles which surround the urethra and support the base of the penis begin to contract rhythmically and regularly. Seminal fluid is forced along the urethra and pumped out of the tip of the penis under pressure. Usually the semen spurts out, although sometimes – particularly in older men or men ejaculating for a second time in quick succession – it may just ooze.

In addition to the ejaculation of semen, powerful reflex contractions of muscles in the abdomen, pelvis and buttocks all contribute to the overall sensation of orgasm.

Resolution phase   For the first few seconds after ejaculation, the glans becomes extremely sensitive and continued stimulation may even be painful. Usually, there is an almost immediate loss of erection, with the penis rapidly returning to half its erect size, before slowly shrinking back to its non-aroused condition. The testicles also decrease to their resting size and are lowered to their normal position.

A pleasant feeling of warmth and total relaxation, with the release of all muscle tension, invariably leads into a deep sleep if you are in a comfortable situation and allow yourself to drift off.

For most men, the resolution phase is also associated with a refractory period, during which the man is unable to become sexually aroused. This may last only a few minutes, or as long as hours, even days. Once a man is over the age of 50, he may only be able to ejaculate once in 24 hours.

Variation in sexual response

A variety of factors, including mood, surroundings and feelings for the partner, can influence the intensity of response at a particular moment. There can also be a wide variation in the timing of the excitement and plateau phases between different individuals and in one man on different occasions.

In addition, ejaculation may not always be the most pleasurable moment. Powerful reflex pelvic muscle contractions occurring either before or after ejaculation can be more satisfying, with ejaculation itself coming as rather an anti-climax!

Dr Bernard Zilbergeld, in his book *Men and Sex*, emphasises that an orgasmic experience can be heightened by learning to relax more during sex, by focusing on bodily sensations and by avoiding the tendency to restrict movements, breathing and noise. Spending more time stimulating your partner during your plateau phase can also enhance your orgasm.

It is important to disregard the popular myth that having reached the plateau phase, you are obliged to go on to orgasm. Although stopping love-making or masturbation at this stage may occasionally cause soreness or discomfort in the testicles, this is not in any way harmful.

·Conception in women

Conception begins with the fertilisation of an ovum (egg) by one of the thousands of sperm that have survived the journey up the woman's vagina, through the cervix and uterus (womb) and into a fallopian tube. The fertilised ovum then has to implant itself successfully within the lining of the uterus for conception to be complete and an embryo to develop into a baby.

Passage of the egg

Around the middle of a woman's menstrual cycle, 14 days before the start of her next menstrual period, an egg is released from one or other ovary. Following ovulation, the egg is drawn into the nearby open end of the fallopian tube to begin its journey towards the uterus.

Rhythmic contractions of the muscles in the fallopian tube wall propel the egg along. It takes about four days for the egg to reach the cavity of the uterus. If it is not fertilised, it breaks up and is lost with the next menstrual period.

Passage of the sperm

Within 30 seconds of ejaculation during unprotected sexual intercourse, several million of the 100 million sperm released will have reached the uterus. Their passage through the cervix is assisted by a combination of the force of ejaculation, reflex contractions of the female pelvic muscles and, most importantly, the powerful swimming motion of the sperm tails.

Those sperm unable to penetrate the mucus barrier across the cervix remain in the vagina and soon die off. In fact, for much of a woman's menstrual cycle, apart from a few days around ovulation, this barrier is of a consistency that usually keeps out all the sperm anyway.

Of the few thousand sperm which survive the swim up the uterus cavity, only a few hundred reach the fallopian tube and have the chance to achieve fertilisation.

Fertilisation

Usually, just one sperm fuses with the egg. As the head of the sperm strikes the outer surface of the egg, a thin cap overlying the sperm's genetic material bursts to release enzymes which assist its penetration of the substance surrounding the ovum's genetic material.

Once the sperm head is fixed, the rest of the sperm becomes detached and, following fusion of the two collections of genetic material, the resulting zygote develops a protective covering to prevent other sperm from penetrating.

The possibility of fertilisation depends on timing, the egg surviving in the upper part of the fallopian tube for a maximum of only 24 hours and sperm surviving for a maximum of seven days inside one of the fallopian tubes. To implant successfully, the zygote normally has to develop for another day or two, through a series of cell divisions, which is why conception is more likely if fertilisation occurs well up the fallopian tube and not too close to the uterus.

However, owing to variations in the time of ovulation and how long the egg and sperm can actually survive, the fertile period may be as long as ten days of the menstrual cycle.

Growing up

The most rapid phase of human body growth and development occurs inside the uterus, from the moment of conception onwards. Initially, body cells proliferate dramatically through a continuous process of cell division, with cell numbers doubling each time the cells divide. Then, as a result of the genetic blueprint in each cell, different body parts and organs begin to take shape. By the end of the first three months of pregnancy, the foetus is recognisable as a tiny human being and all the major organs will have formed. Over the remaining six months the baby grows steadily in size.

Infancy is also a period of rapid body growth, with the baby usually tripling in birth weight over the first year. Height generally increases at a steady rate of 5–8 cm each year after the age of two. In addition to growing taller and heavier, children go through a major change in body proportions, with their trunk and limbs catching up in relation to the size of their head.

Although all the various body organs are present at birth, many of them are immature in terms of both their structure and their function. An important part of early growth and development is therefore a steady maturation of these different organs. For example, most of the brain has grown before birth, but considerable changes in its internal structure, as well as in the rest of the nervous system, are necessary for the development of essential skills. Much of this maturation process involves the formation of new connections between nerves and is dependent on the brain receiving adequate and reliable stimulation through all five senses – touch, smell, taste, sight and hearing.

CONTROL OF GROWTH AND DEVELOPMENT

Both the external and internal body changes that occur as a normal part of growth and development depend primarily on the action of growth hormone, which is produced by the pituitary gland at the base of the brain. Growth hormone stimulates the formation of new protein in most body tissues, speeding up the process of cell proliferation to cause a steady increase in the bulk and complexity of these different structures. Interestingly, the influence of growth hormone on all these cell changes appears to be most marked during sleep.

Changes at puberty

Male puberty is defined as the period of development during which a boy achieves physical sexual maturity and the ability to father children. In contrast, 'adolescence' includes the emotional as well as the physical changes that occur during the transition from boy to man. The start of puberty occurs when the pituitary gland at the base of the brain is stimulated to secrete gonadotrophin hormones. The gonadotrophins step up the production of testosterone by the testicles and within two years the boy will begin to notice the characteristic physical changes of puberty.

Puberty may start at any age from ten years old, but usually the onset is between 12 and 14, taking on average two-and-a-half years to complete. Boys who mature later or at a slower rate are understandably likely to be sensitive or worried about this. However, later maturity has no significance with regard to future virility or fertility.

Some of the changes of puberty generally occur in a predictable sequence, with an increase in the size of the testicles and scrotum being followed by enlargement of the penis. Pubic hair generally appears before armpit hair, with facial hair emerging later.

'WET DREAMS'

Waking up to find a damp, sticky patch of semen on the sheets can be a highly embarrassing experience for a teenage boy. However, this phenomenon of spontaneously ejaculating during the night is perfectly normal and unrelated to any previous sexual experience. Often the boy will be unable to remember actually having an erotic dream.

Spontaneous nocturnal emissions – or 'wet dreams', as they are more popularly known – begin at puberty. They may occur frequently until the boy finds some other regular sexual outlet, either masturbation or intercourse.

The majority of boys have reached about 80 per cent of their adult height before puberty. Nevertheless, there will usually be a noticeable pubertal growth spurt along with all the other changes, which include:

- hair growth on the chest and abdomen
- muscle development, particularly around the upper chest and thighs
- voice breaks (drops to a lower pitch), due to enlargement of the larynx
- sperm production starts in the testicles.

Middle age

After childhood and puberty, the adult years appear to be a period in which nothing much goes on in the body. However, constant activity occurs in body tissues throughout adult life, for example:

- the bones are living tissues that constantly renew their internal structure to remain strong and healthy
- muscle cells grow in size and develop more energy-producing units (mitochondria) if exercised regularly
- skin, intestine lining and blood cells are continuously replaced
- intellectual powers may not peak until a man is in his 30s, or even later.

Growing old

The ageing process, during which body tissues and organs simply wear out, even if they have remained free of disease, normally starts to affect physical and intellectual capacity at some time after the age of 60 and progresses much faster in some men than in others. Ageing remains a mystery to doctors and scientists, although there are several theories as to the exact biological mechanisms involved, for example:

- a progressive decline in the body's immune system means that it is no longer able to defend itself as efficiently against bacteria, viruses and the growth of cancer cells
- a gradual build-up of toxins takes place inside the body
- the DNA templates, which control the copying of individual cells, are worn out, causing mistakes to occur in tissue and organ regeneration.

A number of changes may occur in the body as a normal part of ageing (*see opposite*). These changes are thought to be controlled, at least partly, by the genes you have inherited from your parents. However, a variety of lifestyle factors, such as cigarette-smoking, poor diet, lack of exercise, excessive alcohol consumption and regular exposure to strong sunlight, are known to accelerate the age-related degeneration of body organs and tissues.

Most men can slow down this natural decline by having a healthy lifestyle and remaining physically and intellectually active. Regular physical exercise can help to keep the heart, lungs, bones, muscles and circulation in good condition. Mental agility can often be preserved by ensuring that the brain is regularly stimulated with new ideas and activities.

It is certainly a mistake to regard illness, loss of mobility, loss of independence or the onset of dementia as an inevitable result of growing old; any persistent symptom of ill health should be reported to the doctor.

AGEING PROCESS

As you grow older, you may notice a variety of changes in your body and its performance, including:

- loss of muscle strength, bulk and endurance (stamina)
- increased joint stiffness
- injuries and wounds taking longer to heal
- reduced bone density, with increased risk of fracture
- compression of spinal bones and discs, causing loss of height
- wrinkling of skin, due to collagen degeneration
- increased likelihood of bruising, due to weakened skin capillaries
- impaired lung efficiency, resulting from reduced elasticity
- greying of hair as pigment-producing cells die off
- less efficient processing of alcohol and medication by the liver
- need for reading glasses, due to stiffness in eye lenses
- deafness to high-pitched sounds
- difficulties with short-term memory.

Sexual function in older men

While some older men prefer to cease their love-making, many others want to continue demonstrating love and affection for their partner in a physical way. Unfortunately, many older couples wrongly believe that an active sex life should end at 60 and they feel guilty or ashamed that what they are doing is in some way dirty.

In fact, assuming both partners want to make love, the enjoyment can actually improve in later life once the pressures of work and the worry of unwanted pregnancy have been left behind.

If an older man is having sexual problems, whether physical or psychological, he should start by consulting his doctor. For many of the common difficulties a solution can be found. For example, a change in medication, if relevant, may help improve potency (*see pages 145–7*).

Advice on love-making positions that are less physically stressful can overcome limitations caused by third-age health problems, such as osteoarthritis or angina. Referral to a professional counsellor (*see page 105*) has helped many older couples to resolve their sexual fears and anxieties.

CHAPTER 2

HOW TO STAY PHYSICALLY HEALTHY

MANY different factors determine whether you will remain physically healthy throughout your life. Some of the influences are clearly beyond your control, such as the genes you have inherited from your parents, the food you were given as a child, exposure to infection and whether you received all the recommended immunisations. However, many aspects of the way you live also affect your physical condition.

By adopting a healthy lifestyle, being aware of specific risks to your physical health and alert to the possible early-warning symptoms of illness, you will not only reduce your chances of dying young, you should also be able to enjoy a better quality of life well into old age.

Decisions you make about your diet, how much exercise you take and habits such as smoking and drinking alcohol can all directly harm or benefit your long-term physical health. You also need to know which symptoms to report to your doctor, how to keep an eye out for early-warning signs of disease through regular self-examination of different parts of your body and also when you should have the various screening tests designed to detect hidden diseases. Immunisation and accident prevention are also vitally important.

Diet and nutrition

A healthy diet

We need food to provide the energy that keeps our body cells alive and active. We also need food to supply the raw materials used for the growth, maintenance and repair of all the body's tissues and organs.

However, eating is also an important part of our social lives and should therefore be a source of pleasure, not anxiety.

Unfortunately, since we became aware that diet can influence health, we have been bombarded with stories about the nutritional qualities of different products, most of these resulting from the food industry's desire to sell particular brands.

Healthy eating does not mean giving up all your favourite meals, nor spending hours studying the nutrient and calorie content of hundreds of different foods. The key to a healthy diet is simply variation and balance, with the emphasis on extending rather than restricting the range of foods you normally eat.

Variation and balance

To satisfy all your nutritional requirements by consuming the recommended intake of each vitamin and mineral and the correct mixture of carbohydrates, fats and proteins (*see Glossary*), you should try to eat as wide a variety of foods as possible. The easiest way to do this is to choose a range of foods each day from each of the five major food groups:

- breads, cereals and other grain products, such as rice
- fruits
- vegetables
- dairy produce, such as milk, cheese and yogurt
- plant proteins, such as dried beans, peas, nuts and seeds, and/or animal protein from eggs, fish, poultry or meat.

As well as having a balanced diet, healthy eating also means not taking in too much of any one kind of food and avoiding a surplus of calories, which will cause an increase in body weight. The ideal diet supplies sufficient calories to fulfil the body's energy requirements, which obviously depends on how much energy is being burned up through physical activity that day (*see page 64*). To achieve a healthy supply of both calories and nutrients, the recommended proportions of energy provided by carbohydrates, fats and proteins are 50–55 per cent, less than 30 per cent and about 15 per cent respectively.

Many men consume much more fat than this recommended intake. Also, most of the carbohydrate foods they eat contain predominantly refined sugars that tend to be high in calories, but low in fibre, vitamins and minerals. A high intake of fats, particularly saturated fats, raises blood cholesterol and increases the risk of heart disease. Too much fat, too many refined carbohydrates and too much alcohol (particularly beer or lager) are the reasons why so many men in the UK are overweight. Heavy consumption of sugar also encourages tooth decay.

Not eating enough fibre or drinking insufficient water can interfere with the efficiency of the digestive system, causing, for example, constipation and other bowel disorders.

To achieve a balanced diet, in addition to eating a wide variety of foods, you should therefore increase your fibre intake, cut down on fat and eat fewer sugary foods.

More fibre

A high intake of fibre is essential, not only to prevent constipation but also to help control the absorption of glucose (sugar) and digested fats from the intestine into the circulation. People who eat sufficient fibre are less likely to develop an abnormally high blood cholesterol level and less likely to suffer sudden changes in their blood sugar level, which can cause a variety of unpleasant symptoms such as headaches, dizziness and fatigue.

High-fibre foods fill you up without adding a lot of calories to your diet. Foods rich in fibre include wholegrain bread and cereal, fresh fruits and vegetables, brown rice and dried beans.

Less sugar

Foods packed with refined sugars, such as cakes, biscuits and jam, provide calories but are lacking in essential nutrients. In excess, they increase the risk of obesity and tooth decay. It is important to remember that many canned products, including certain brands of soup, baked beans, vegetables and fruits, contain a lot of added sugar, as does ketchup, because sugar is often used as a food preservative.

Easy ways to cut down your sugar intake are to pick unsweetened or artificially sweetened products, drink low-calorie soft drinks or water and avoid adding sugar to tea or coffee.

Less fat

To reduce the risk of obesity and heart disease, no more than 30 per cent of your energy intake should come from fat. Also, when you are eating or cooking with fat, try to choose unsaturated rather than saturated fats whenever possible.

Saturated fat, which is found in meat, milk, cheese and butter and which is added to many processed foods, is converted in the liver to cholesterol. A build-up of cholesterol results in the walls of the arteries furring up with deposits of fat. Unsaturated fats, found in oily fish, nuts, margarine and most types of vegetable oil, do not increase cholesterol production and are thought to have a protective effect on the heart and blood vessels.

To keep your fat intake down:

- eat lean meats such as chicken (without the skin), fish, liver and kidney
- limit your consumption of processed meats
- trim off the visible fat before cooking meat
- bulk out red meat dishes with a vegetable protein, such as red kidney beans
- cut down on fried food, and always use a polyunsaturated vegetable oil when you do fry
- use low-fat spreads and cheeses
- drink skimmed rather than whole milk
- eat a maximum of four eggs each week – they are rich in cholesterol
- when you eat out, remember that sauces, gravies and dressings are usually full of fat
- avoid puddings and pastries, which are also loaded with fat.

Less salt

Most people eat far more salt than they need. In some individuals this may be a factor in the development of abnormally high blood pressure. Anyone with high blood pressure or heart failure is usually advised to cut down their salt intake because it can make both these disorders worse.

To limit the amount of salty foods you eat:

- avoid processed foods which contain a lot of salt, such as certain canned vegetables, soups and ketchups
- don't add salt (or add less) to your cooking and don't put salt on your food at the table
- beware pickles, chutneys, sausages, bacon, beefburgers, and some cheeses and butters which have a high salt content
- use a salt substitute – but not in excess.

Healthy eating habits

It is not just what you eat but also the way you eat your food that can influence your health. Eating virtually nothing during the day and then a large meal late in the evening, for example, is a common reason for putting on weight. Your body's metabolism works more efficiently on a regular supply of food energy. Starving yourself just causes the chemical activities in the cells that burn up calories to switch off. Also, you should take time out to rest and relax during and for at least half an hour after a meal and avoid vigorous exercise for up to three hours. Otherwise, you are likely to end up with indigestion, heartburn or wind.

Choosing a healthy snack

Unfortunately, a lot of the popular convenience foods, which are either ready to eat or quick and easy to prepare, do not meet the requirements for a healthy diet. They tend to be high in calories and contain a lot of saturated fat plus added sugar or salt; they are also usually low in fibre and short on essential nutrients. While the occasional unhealthy snack will not do any harm, eaten regularly this type of food increases your chance of becoming overweight and deficient in certain vitamins and minerals.

Many healthy and nutritious convenience foods are now available. It is a good idea before buying, therefore, to check the label for the fat, sugar and salt content. Also, remember that glucose, fructose, maltose and caramel are just different sorts of sugar.

Rather than snacking on crisps, cakes, biscuits and sweets, it is better to chew on a piece of fresh fruit or a raw vegetable like a carrot. If you make a sandwich, use wholegrain bread and a low-fat spread, then choose a lean filling such as low-fat cottage cheese or tuna.

Fast foods, like most convenience foods, also tend to be high in calories, saturated fat and salt, and low in fibre. Although they do provide many essential nutrients, including protein, some vitamins and minerals, fast foods are often lacking in vitamin A, vitamin C and calcium. When ordering fast food, watch out for the high-fat, calorie-rich sauces that often accompany a burger. And, even though chicken and fish are leaner meats than beef, when they are served as fast food they are generally fried in fat-rich batter. To balance the meal, have a side-salad without dressing and choose water rather than a carbonated soft drink.

Nutritional needs throughout life

A range of nutrients which must be present in the diet to maintain good health has been identified. For most of these vitamins and minerals, a recommended daily intake has been calculated, which represents the average quantity of that nutrient which each person should consume every day. This should satisfy the nutritional needs of around 97 per cent of the population without overdosing those who actually require less.

TABLE 1
Reference Nutrient Intakes (RNIs) – daily recommended consumption for adult males (19–50 years)

Vitamin A	0.7mg
Thiamine	1.0mg
Riboflavin	1.3mg
Niacin	17mg
Pantothenic acid	No recommendation – deficiency unknown
Vitamin B$_6$	1.4mg
Vitamin B$_{12}$	1.5mcg
Biotin	No RNI (suggested daily intake 10–200mcg)
Folic acid	200mcg
Vitamin C	40mg
Vitamin D	No RNI between 4 and 65 years
Vitamin E	No recommendation (suggested daily intake of alphatocopherol 3–4mg)
Vitamin K	1mcg per kg body weight
Calcium	700mg
Iodine	140mcg
Iron	8.7mg
Magnesium	300mg
Potassium	3.5g
Selenium	75mcg
Zinc	9.5mg
Phosphorus	550mg
Sodium	1.6g
Chloride	2.5g
Copper	1.2mg

These figures, known as Reference Nutrient Intakes (RNIs), which have replaced the old units of nutritional value, Recommended Daily Amounts (RDAs), are tabulated opposite for adult males aged between 19 and 50 years. Each RNI is a recommendation for the whole of this group of men, but it will not be exactly correct for all of them. This is because other factors, such as lifestyle and the state of a person's health, influence nutrient requirements. However, if your intake of a nutrient is well below its RNI, there is certainly a risk of developing symptoms of deficiency.

To reduce the risk of illness as you get older and to boost your recovery after an illness, it is essential to continue to eat a healthy diet. It may also be necessary to adapt your eating habits to compensate for changes in your body that occur as a normal part of the ageing process.

TABLE 2
Common nutrient deficiencies in elderly men

Nutrient	Cause of deficiency (in addition to low intake)	Food source
Iron	Reduced absorption from ageing digestive system	Wholegrain cereals, green leafy vegetables, liver, fish and meat
Thiamine	Ageing increases requirement	Wholegrain bread and cereals, brown rice, beans, nuts, fish and liver
Calcium	Reduced absorption from ageing digestive system	Green leafy vegetables, dairy produce, eggs and fish with edible bones
Vitamin D	Lack of sunlight if housebound	Eggs, margarine and oily fish (sardines, tuna and herring)
Vitamin C	Lack of and overcooking vegetables and fruit	Fresh vegetables and fruit (particularly citrus)

Although older men usually continue to eat a sufficient amount of food, their diet is typically lacking in variety and balance, particularly for those men living alone who cook for themselves. They often start to rely on processed or convenience foods, which are a lot easier to buy and prepare, but may cost more than fresh products.

Some of the more common nutrient deficiencies found in elderly men are listed on page 63, with advice on which foods should be eaten to prevent or correct each of these deficiencies.

Calorie requirements in men

Your body needs a certain amount of energy from food (measured in calories) to maintain vital physical and chemical functions both at rest and during exercise, to keep itself warm and also to build and repair different tissues, such as bone and muscle. For most healthy men, average daily calorie requirements are calculated from age and general level of physical activity (*see Table A*). The number of calories burned up per hour by the average man taking part in a variety of different activities has also been measured (*see Table B*). With this information, you should be able to work out roughly the calories you need to suit your particular requirements.

TABLE A
Average calorie requirements for men

Age	Lifestyle	Calories/day
18–35 years	Inactive	2,500
	Active	3,000
	Very active	3,500
36–70 years	Inactive	2,400
	Active	2,900
	Very active	3,400
70+ years	Inactive	2,200
	Active	2,500

Note These are average values; there are a few people who have a slow metabolism and therefore require less food energy to keep their body running. Also, there are a few 'fast burners' who do not put on weight even though eating large amounts of calories.

Men who consistently consume more calories than they need for their daily physical activity and body maintenance requirements will inevitably put on weight. Surplus food is converted into fat, which is then deposited around the body, particularly the abdomen, where it forms the familiar paunch.

TABLE B
Calorie consumption per hour of activity

Activity	Calories burned
Sleeping	65
Writing	100
Walking	250
Brisk walking	300
Cycling	300
Slow running	400
Swimming	500
Squash	650
Fast running	650

Note Some of these values clearly depend on the amount of effort put in, for example, swimming would burn 500 calories/hour only if you were doing continuous lengths of the pool.

Calorie needs in older men
As the body ages, its energy requirements decrease. One reason is the tendency to take less vigorous exercise in later life. In addition, a progressive reduction in the basal metabolic rate (the energy used by the body to maintain vital functions, such as breathing and heartbeat) occurs as a normal part of the ageing process. This explains why older men may put on weight unless they adjust their eating and exercise habits.

Nutrient supplements

Most men obtain the recommended amounts (*see page 62*) of vitamins and minerals simply by eating a varied and balanced diet. If you eat the sort of healthy diet described earlier, taking a supplement is unlikely to make any significant difference to your health.

However, anyone who eats a lot of processed or highly refined foods runs the risk of becoming marginally deficient in a variety of nutrients, including vitamins B₆ and E, chromium, zinc, copper and selenium. A lot of vague symptoms and minor skin problems are thought to be due to a marginal deficiency in one or more nutrients, but this can only be confirmed by a doctor arranging specific blood tests.

A variety of other conditions or situations can also lead to vitamin or mineral deficiency:

- elderly men often neglect their diet for the reasons described earlier
- men struggling with poverty, alcoholism, drug abuse and mental illness are all likely to have an inadequate diet
- chronic diseases of the stomach, intestine, pancreas or liver may interfere with either the absorption or digestion of a particular nutrient; kidney failure can lead to a deficiency of potassium, magnesium, calcium and vitamin D
- long-term medication may upset the absorption or metabolism of a specific nutrient: for example, some anti-epilepsy drugs increase the need for folic acid and vitamin D
- a drastic weight-reducing diet, in which there is a low intake of food or limitations on the types of food being eaten, can be inadequate nutritionally.

How to choose a supplement

It is best to consult your doctor before starting to take any nutrient supplement. Products which contain only one type of vitamin or mineral may cause problems by increasing the body's demand for other nutrients. Multi-vitamin and mineral preparations contain a variety of nutrients in different doses and combinations, which can be confusing.

Some brands of supplement contain several times the recommended daily dose of a nutrient, which in certain circumstances could lead to unpleasant adverse effects. Too much of a vitamin or mineral can do more harm than good. For example, in large amounts:

- vitamin B₆ (pyridoxine) may damage nerves, causing numbness, pins and needles and weakness
- vitamin D may cause nausea, vomiting and muscle spasm
- vitamin A may result in skin irritation and hair loss
- iron may upset the digestive system, leading to diarrhoea or constipation.

An unhealthy diet cannot be made healthy by taking a nutrient supplement. The right mixture of foods in a balanced diet provides not only the required vitamins and minerals, but also the correct proportion of fat, protein, carbohydrate and fibre.

Losing weight

An accurate way to assess whether you are carrying too much weight is to calculate your Body Mass Index (BMI). This figure is derived by dividing your weight, measured in kilograms, by the square of your height, measured in metres (BMI = W/H^2). For example, a man who weighs 83kg and is 1.83m tall would have a BMI of 24.78 (i.e. 83 ÷ [1.83 x 1.83]).

If your BMI is between 20 and 25, this is considered healthy. However, a BMI between 25 and 30 is a sign of being overweight, and over 30 is defined as obese. At least 30 per cent of men in the UK are overweight and almost 5 per cent are in the obese category.

Overweight men tend to have less energy, they are more likely to become overheated and breathless during exercise, their ankles are more likely to swell and the joints in their back and legs are more likely to ache. Overweight and obese men are more vulnerable to:

- high blood pressure
- high blood cholesterol
- gallstones
- varicose veins
- osteoarthritis
- coronary heart disease
- diabetes
- stroke.

Weight-reducing diets

Most men who are overweight are not suffering from any hormonal or metabolic disorder, they simply have a calorie intake that consistently exceeds their energy requirements. This is usually due to a combination of over-eating and not taking enough exercise to burn off the excess calories.

Tackling the problem of over-eating is as difficult for most men as giving up smoking or cutting down on alcohol. The fact that no single diet is universally successful is reflected by the large numbers of popular diet books on sale, each recommending different types of diet. However, basic principles of successful weight reduction are:

- first set yourself a realistic target weight and aim to lose about a kilogram each week
- consider joining a slimming group to help keep you motivated
- choose a varied, balanced diet (as described earlier) – the sort of diet that you can follow as a normal part of your life
- eat two to three proper small meals, don't miss out a meal and don't snack in between; if you must snack, choose healthy foods
- increase your intake of fibre-rich, starchy foods, such as potatoes, rice and pasta (with a tomato-based rather than creamy sauce)
- cut down on refined, sugary foods
- eat less fat, particularly saturated fat
- cut down on alcohol (particularly beer and lager), switch to low-calorie soft drinks and drink plenty of water
- eat slowly and cut up your food into small pieces so that it takes longer to eat; use a smaller plate
- don't eat while you are reading or watching TV.

When you achieve your target weight, it is important not to slip back into your previous unhealthy eating habits. Unfortunately, many men often end up weighing more than they did before they originally started to diet. This cycle of weight loss followed by weight gain is now thought to be more damaging to physical health than remaining consistently overweight.

EXERCISE

Losing weight is not just about diet and healthy nutrition: regular strenuous exercise is also important. Brisk walking, swimming and cycling are all good activities to burn up extra calories and reduce your body's fat stores. Regular physical activity also raises your basal metabolic rate (see *Glossary*), so that you burn up more calories at rest. Also, a vigorous workout can depress appetite and take your mind off the urge to snack.

Warning Consult your doctor before beginning any exercise programme if you are overweight.

Sports nutrition

It is a common misconception that if you play a lot of sport or train hard you need to take some form of nutrient supplement. Although it is true that the more active a man is, the higher his calorie intake should be, just eating a varied balanced diet should satisfy the body's demand for all the different vitamins, minerals, amino acids and other nutrients. Taking a supplement will not normally make any difference to physical fitness, nor to the speed of recovery after intense training or an injury.

Try to eat at least three hours before you exercise. If you eat less than an hour before, you are likely to feel nauseous and uncomfortable because food is still in your stomach. If you haven't eaten for more than five hours, there is a good chance you could develop abdominal discomfort or feel light-headed.

The best type of food to eat if you plan to exercise later is starchy carbohydrate, such as pasta or potatoes. In contrast with fat- and protein-rich foods, such as steak, carbohydrates are digested and absorbed quickly to provide an immediate supply of energy for the muscle cells in the form of glucose (sugar).

Drink enough fluids

Body water is lost when you perspire during strenuous exercise. It is therefore important to drink enough fluids before and after exercise to avoid becoming dehydrated. In hot and humid conditions, or if you are involved in an activity that lasts longer than 45 minutes, it is a good idea to drink small amounts of liquid at regular intervals throughout the exercise.

Feeling thirsty is not a reliable guide to how much fluid you need, so get into the habit of drinking liquids as a normal part of your exercise routine. A good example of fluid replacement being taken seriously is the professional tennis player who drinks something on virtually every changeover. Water is the best drink to prevent dehydration during exercise. Have one or two glasses about half an hour before you start to make sure your tissues begin with a good supply of fluid. If you break off for a rest period after 30–45 minutes, drink another glass. For a continuous activity lasting longer than one hour, such as running a marathon or playing tennis, drink at regular intervals but take only small amounts.

These precautions should prevent the onset of dehydration, which might otherwise spoil both your enjoyment and your performance. Once the exercise is over, drink yet more water, particularly if you have been perspiring heavily.

A high-energy sports drink containing sugar may help keep your muscles supplied with glucose during an endurance event lasting two hours or more, such as running a marathon. However, it is not needed for most sporting activities and there is no scientific evidence to prove that a sports drink actually boosts performance.

A Food Commission report expressed concern at the large amounts of added sugar in sports drinks. One serving of some of the more popular brands provides the equivalent of between eight and 24 lumps of sugar, which is certainly not part of a healthy diet – however many calories you intend to burn up. It is also possible that this high sugar content could encourage dehydration by drawing water out of the bloodstream into the stomach to dilute the drink.

Coffee, tea and cola drinks containing caffeine are best avoided because caffeine acts as a diuretic, which removes more body water in the urine. Although caffeine in high doses is believed to have a stimulant effect on exercise performance, you would need to take it as a concentrated tablet to achieve any benefit, and such a large amount is regarded as a prohibited drug in most sports. Remember also that alcohol is a diuretic which diverts more body water into the urine, increasing the chance of dehydration. You should therefore delay drinking alcohol after exercise until you have restored your body fluids with water.

Salt tablets

Salt replacement is needed only if you are taking part in a long strenuous activity in a hot or humid environment and you are having to drink large amounts of fluid to stay hydrated. Under normal circumstances your body is able to compensate for the salt lost in sweat simply by reducing the amount of salt passed out in the urine.

There is a tendency to blame cramp on lack of salt, but the real reason is more likely to be muscle fatigue or injury. In fact, taking salt tablets when you don't need them may actually bring on an attack of cramp.

Exercise and keeping fit

First, it is important not to confuse good health with good fitness. Rarely being ill does not automatically imply that you are in good physical condition. Likewise, being physically fit is not the same as sporting excellence – you don't have to train for hours in order to improve and maintain your fitness. Rather than visiting a gym or buying special equipment, one easy way to increase the amount of exercise you take is to walk or cycle part of the way to work.

A basic definition of fitness is the ability to cope easily with the physical workload of normal daily activities, without becoming unduly breathless or exhausted, and still have extra energy in reserve to meet any sudden unexpected demand: for example, to be able to carry heavy bags and run for the bus. Your general level of fitness is determined by the efficiency of your heart, lungs, circulation and muscles, which in turn is influenced by how regularly you exercise in a sustained and vigorous way.

Starting a fitness programme

Before starting any strenuous physical activity to get fit, it is advisable to have a check-up from your doctor first if:

- you are over 35 and have done very little exercise for a few years
- you are over 60 years old
- you are significantly overweight
- you are a smoker
- someone in your immediate family developed heart disease before the age of 40
- you are under medical treatment or supervision for high blood pressure, a heart condition, diabetes or any other long-term disease.

These precautions allow your doctor to detect any disorder that could make over-exerting yourself dangerous and to advise which exercises are suitable in your particular circumstances.

Having made the decision to start and been given the go-ahead by your doctor (if necessary), you then need to devise your own fitness programme. Ideally, this should include a mixture of exercises designed to improve all three components of your fitness: endurance, strength and flexibility.

71

When you first begin exercising, don't try to push yourself too hard too soon. Your routine should make you a little breathless, but not gasping for air; tired, but not completely exhausted. Slowly, over a period of several weeks, increase the amount of time and effort you put in as your level of fitness improves.

Strength

Strength is the ability to use muscle force to lift, carry, push or pull a heavy load. Your body contains over 600 muscles to enable it to perform hundreds of different movements. Depending on your build, this muscle tissue may represent anything between one-quarter and one-half of your body weight. If your muscles are weak and out of condition, any activity for which strength is important will be more difficult to perform.

An easy way to assess your muscle strength is to count how many sit-ups you can perform in one minute. It is important to keep your knees bent to avoid straining your lower back and your hands against the side of your head, not behind as this can strain the neck. Around 20–25 sit-ups is average for men under the age of 50; much less than this and you need to strengthen your abdominal muscles.

Flexibility

Flexibility is the ability to stretch, bend or twist through a wide range of movements. This is determined by the degree of suppleness of your joints and the elasticity of your muscles and tendons. A lack of flexibility increases the risk of a sprain or strain resulting from a sudden or violent movement. Tight back and leg muscles can lead to back pain and stiffness after exercise.

To measure your flexibility, try the following sit and reach test. Sitting on the floor with your legs slightly apart and keeping your back and knees straight, lean forward slowly from your waist. If you are unable to get close to touching your heels, you may benefit from stretching exercises to improve the flexibility of your back and hamstring muscles (see flexibility exercises, *pages 76–7*).

Endurance

Endurance is the ability to keep on exercising without stopping to rest. Good endurance depends on the efficiency and performance of your heart, lungs, muscles and circulation. Anyone whose endurance is low will develop muscle fatigue and loss of co-ordination during prolonged exercise, increasing the risk of sustaining an injury.

To test your own endurance level, try walking briskly or jogging for about a mile or, alternatively, walk at a steady pace up three flights of stairs. If you have to stop during this activity to catch your breath, or because your legs are aching, or you end up too breathless to talk properly, you would benefit from exercises to enhance your endurance.

Checking the fitness of your heart

You can check the fitness of your heart by first counting your resting pulse and then measuring your pulse recovery 30 seconds after a session of strenuous exercise. To take your pulse, press your fingertips firmly against the artery on the front of your wrist at the base of your thumb. Count the number of beats over a 15-second period and multiply by four to calculate your heart rate per minute.

The most reliable reading of your resting pulse is the one taken when you have just woken up in the morning. In general, a fit heart is associated with a slow, strong and regular pulse. Men have a slightly higher resting pulse than women, and the values increase a little with age. The table below shows the approximate relationship for men between age, resting pulse and fitness level.

TABLE 3
Resting pulse rates in men

	Age	20–29	30–39	40–49	50+
Fitness	Excellent	≤59	≤63	≤65	≤67
level	Good	60–69	64–71	66–73	68–75
	Fair	70–85	72–85	74–89	76–89
	Poor	≥86	≥86	≥90	≥90

Note If your resting pulse is 100 beats/minute or more, see your doctor as soon as possible.

Step-ups are the easiest type of strenuous exercise to perform indoors. Using a stair or stool about 20cm high, step up and down off it moving one foot after the other. Continue the exercise for at least three minutes at a rate of around 24 step-ups per minute. Then,

73

after 30 seconds' rest check your pulse at the wrist. This time count over a 10-second period only and multiply the figure by six to calculate your heart rate per minute; any longer would allow the pulse to recover further. The table below shows the approximate relationship for men between age, pulse recovery at 30 seconds and fitness level.

TABLE 4
Pulse recovery in men at 30 seconds

	Age	20–29	30–39	40–49	50+
Fitness	Excellent	74	78	80	82
level	Good	76–84	80–86	82–88	84–90
	Fair	86–100	88–100	90–104	92–104
	Poor	>102	>102	>106	>106

Warning Do not perform step-ups if your starting pulse is 100 or over and stop this exercise at once if you develop any symptoms of heart strain (*see pages 78–9*).

How to stay motivated
The benefits to your future health from keeping fit are soon lost if you don't continue to exercise regularly. Unfortunately, as many as 50 per cent of the men who start themselves on an exercise programme drop out within six months. Here are a few tips to help you stay motivated:

- set yourself short-term as well as long-term fitness goals that are not beyond your capabilities
- write down what you hope to achieve, e.g. losing a few kilograms in weight or being able to run for the bus again
- find an exercise partner so you can encourage each other
- choose activities you enjoy and find convenient to do
- vary your routine to avoid becoming bored
- have regular exercise slots at the same time in your weekly schedule
- keep a record of the type and amount of exercise you have been doing so you can monitor your progress
- during a repetitive exercise, count backwards from your target number to zero.

Endurance exercises

To improve your endurance, you need to participate in aerobic activities regularly, i.e. any form of prolonged exercise that can be performed continuously for at least 12 minutes. During aerobic exercise, the heart and lungs work hard enough to maintain a sufficient supply of oxygen to the muscles, allowing the muscle cells to continue functioning normally for a long period. Aerobic activities include jogging, brisk walking, skipping, swimming, dancing and cycling. Regular aerobic exercise carried out for around 20 minutes at a time, three times a week, enhances endurance by boosting the efficiency of your heart, lungs, muscles and circulation.

Target heart rate

To gauge how hard you need to work during aerobic activities to achieve the maximum benefit, you should aim to raise your pulse as near as possible to your target heart rate. When you first start a fitness programme, you are likely to find it impossible to reach this target without breaking the guidelines on not pushing yourself too hard.

Your target heart rate is the sum of your resting pulse plus half the difference between your resting pulse and the theoretical maximum pulse for your age. This theoretical maximum pulse is calculated by subtracting your age from 220. For example, a man of 40 with a resting pulse of 80 has a theoretical maximum pulse of 220 minus 40 which equals 180. Fifty per cent of the difference between his resting pulse and theoretical maximum is 180 minus 80, divided by two, which equals 50. Added to the resting pulse, 80 plus 50, produces a target heart rate of 130 beats per minute. To see how near you are to your target, take your pulse after a few minutes of aerobic activity. Count over a 10-second period and then multiply by six, otherwise your heart will have time to start slowing down again.

Strength exercises

Muscle-strengthening exercises will improve your body shape and posture by increasing muscle tone. They will also make it easier to move heavy loads. There are various types of strength exercises, including:

Multiple repetitions   using small weights to improve muscle strength and tone, without significantly increasing muscle bulk. Start with weights light enough for you to be able to perform at least eight repetitions. Once you can cope easily with 12 repetitions in a minute, move on to a slightly heavier weight. It is important to perform each movement correctly, holding the weight at the furthest point for a count of two and breathing out at the same time. Leave a five-minute gap between each set of repetitions working a particular muscle group and rotate through a circuit of other muscle groups in the meantime. Three circuits of these different exercises are recommended for each workout.

Lifting heavy weights is the way to build up muscle bulk, performing just a few repetitions for each group of muscles because the exercise will be anaerobic (short, sharp bursts of vigorous muscle activity which result in a build-up of lactic acid because the cells need more oxygen than can be supplied). The increase in bulk is due to the formation of more contracting strands inside each muscle fibre, making the fibre thicker, but there is no change in the actual number of muscle fibres.

Isometric exercises contract the muscle fibres, but without changing the length of the muscle, so there is no visible movement in that part of the body. This can be done either by holding part of the body in a fixed position against the pull of gravity, or by using one group of muscles to resist an attempted movement in another. These static exercises which boost tone and strength are unsuitable for anyone who has had a heart condition or stroke because they tend to raise blood pressure.

To reduce the risk of injury, always warm up with gentle stretching and loosening-up movements before starting any muscle-strengthening exercises. While it is usual for strength exercises to cause some burning discomfort, stop at once if you notice a sharp pain which could signal injury. Strength exercises are best done in a properly equipped gym supervised by an experienced instructor. Children under the age of 14 should not be lifting heavy weights as a growing skeleton is more vulnerable to injury.

Flexibility exercises
Exercises to maintain and improve flexibility will help posture, counteract the generalised aches and stiffness associated with a

sedentary lifestyle and reduce the chance of injury if you have to make a sudden or extreme movement. A range of stretching exercises should be carried out before or after any vigorous physical activity as part of warming up and cooling down (*see over*). Stretching exercises are also important if you are doing a regular muscle-strengthening programme as this training tends to tighten and shorten the muscles.

When you stretch, never bounce or jerk the muscle and never force the movement to a point where it becomes painful. Stretch until you feel a pull and hold this position for a count of ten. The most important muscle stretches involve the calf muscles, the front and back of the thighs, the front of the hips, the lower part of the back and the muscles across the chest and shoulders.

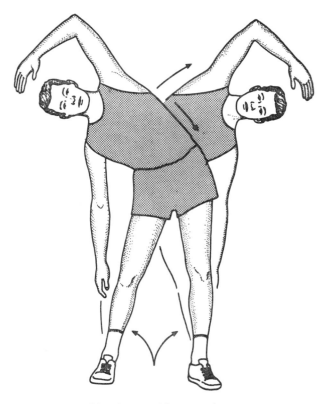

Muscle-stretching exercise

Exercising safely

Anyone who exercises or plays sport regularly is bound to pick up the occasional minor injury. However, while some of these injuries may be due to external causes beyond your control, such as foul play, many could be prevented by taking certain precautions, for example:

- always use the protective equipment available for a specific sport
- replace exercise shoes that have become excessively worn, or which no longer fit properly
- warm up with a routine of stretching and loosening-up exercises for at least ten minutes before the activity – this makes the tissues more elastic and therefore less vulnerable to injury
- cool down with muscle stretches and by continuing to move around for a few minutes after the activity to remove lactic acid from the muscles and thereby reduce subsequent stiffness and soreness
- make sure that playing equipment, such as the handle on a racket or the grip on an oar, is the correct size for you to reduce the chance of a repetitive strain injury
- avoid alcohol or any drug that might make you feel dizzy or drowsy: the resultant loss of co-ordination or delay in reaction time could lead to an injury
- iron out any problems in your technique by consulting a coach or a coaching manual; many injuries are due to basic errors in the way a movement is performed.

An injury that remains painful, tender, stiff or swollen needs further treatment; otherwise, there is a risk of either making the injury worse or developing a second injury by trying to protect the first. Finally, an essential part of exercising safely is to be aware of warning symptoms that suggest you are overworking or damaging part of your body. Pain, soreness or stiffness in your muscles before you start an activity suggests that you should be allowing yourself a longer recovery time between training or playing sessions. Pain, stiffness or swelling in your joints could be the result of excessive jarring because you are not wearing cushioned insoles inside your exercise shoes.

Danger signals that you might be overtaxing your heart during strenuous exercise include:

- chest pain or pain in the neck or arms
- palpitations or skipped heart beats

- nausea, dizziness, light-headedness or feeling faint
- severe breathlessness
- extreme fatigue.

Stop exercising at once if you suffer any of the above symptoms while you are exercising and have a check-up from your doctor before continuing with your fitness programme.

Exercise and illness

Although there are a few acute medical conditions for which exercise is not recommended, such as infection and anaemia, with most chronic illnesses it is important to remain as physically active as possible. Participating in some form of regular exercise will often help minimise the amount of disability resulting from a particular disorder, as well as reducing the risk of developing complications. Even with diseases for which exercise does not have any direct benefit, staying active is still important to prevent the steady deterioration in general health that occurs with a progressive loss of fitness. Continuing to exercise is also good for morale.

If you have a chronic disorder such as asthma, diabetes, high blood pressure or arthritis, it is essential to see your doctor for a check-up and to obtain advice on which activities you can safely take part in before starting a fitness programme.

Even men who are confined to bed or a wheelchair can benefit from a regular routine of stretching and loosening-up exercises.

WARNING – EXERCISE AND INFECTION

Do not be tempted to continue exercising when you have symptoms of an infection, such as a sore throat, fever, swollen glands or a mucus-producing cough. Not only will your performance be below par, but with some viral infections, strenuous exercise can result in a dangerous complication, like myocarditis (inflammation of the heart).

Body care

Skin, nails and hair

An important part of staying physically healthy is to take good care of your skin, nails and hair. If you look good, you are also likely to feel good. Eating a balanced, varied diet, as described earlier, and drinking sufficient amounts of water during the day will help keep your skin, hair and nails in good condition. It is also important, however, not to neglect these parts of your body through inadequate personal care or other unhealthy habits.

Skin-care tips

- make sure your diet contains plenty of fresh fruit and vegetables
- drink at least eight glasses of water every day
- give up smoking as this encourages premature wrinkling
- wash regularly with a mild soap and water to remove dirt and dead skin
- rinse off all soap thoroughly
- do not spend too long in the bath or shower and make sure that the water is not too hot
- use a moisturiser each time you wash if you suffer from dry skin
- dry carefully between your fingers and toes
- cover up with tightly woven, cotton clothing when you are out in the sun; put a sunscreen with a high protection factor on any exposed skin; also, wear a wide-brimmed hat
- wrap up well in cold, windy weather
- avoid direct contact with irritant substances, such as household cleaners and cement, by wearing protective gloves.

Nail-care tips

- don't cut your nails too short
- cut your toenails straight across to stop them ingrowing
- soften your nails in warm water before cutting them
- to protect against nail infection, wear rubber gloves when your hands are being continually immersed in water
- see a doctor if your nails become discoloured or start to crumble as this could be due to a fungal infection.

Hair-care tips

- shampoo your hair regularly to remove any build-up of dirt and grease
- massage your scalp to stimulate blood flow and relax tension
- rinse hair thoroughly under a shower stream if possible
- use a conditioner to smooth the outer surface of the hairs
- keep the hairdryer at least 15cm away to avoid heat damage
- leave your hair slightly damp
- don't brush your hair when it is wet, use a wide-toothed comb; hair is at its weakest when wet
- avoid over-vigorous rubbing of wet hair, which can cause split ends and tangling
- beware of using harsh anti-dandruff shampoos – ask your barber or hairdresser for advice on a suitable preparation.

Looking after your feet

Much of the advice on foot care relates to the prevention of athlete's foot, which is covered in detail in **Chapter 6**. In addition:

- use a pumice stone to remove dead skin from the heels and balls of your feet
- discard shoes that are worn beyond repair, or no longer fit properly
- wear natural materials, such as cotton socks and leather shoes, to reduce sweating. If you suffer from smelly feet, wear insoles made of activated charcoal, which absorb sweat and odour particles
- change socks daily to prevent foot odour – a powder containing an antibacterial drug to reduce the numbers of skin bacteria and an antioxidant to slow down the chemical breakdown of sweat can also help
- if you develop a foot problem, such as a corn, callus or bunion, see a member of the Society of Chiropodists★ (who will have the qualification SRCh) or a member of the British Chiropody Association★.

Eye-care tips

It is important to have a routine eye test at least every two years, or sooner if you notice any change in your vision (*see pages 197–9*). Your sight is precious and irreplaceable, so take good care of your eyes:

- use eye protection if you work with dangerous chemicals or high-speed machinery
- have a light shining on to the page when you are reading or writing, preferably from behind one of your shoulders
- rest your eyes frequently during close work, particularly when using a VDU, by staring into space for a few seconds every 15 minutes to prevent eye strain
- when watching TV, sit at least five feet from the screen
- wear sunglasses in strong sunlight to cut down glare
- a tinted visor is essential when welding as the intense light can damage the eyes.
- fit spectacles worn for sport with plastic lenses, otherwise switch to contact lenses
- wear protective goggles to play squash
- wear goggles to help prevent eye irritation if you are swimming in a highly chlorinated pool
- avoid rubbing your eyes as this is a common way of picking up infection
- ask your pharmacist to recommend eye drops or an eye bath for tired, dry or sore eyes, but if the discomfort persists have your eyes checked by an optician or doctor.

Taking care of teeth and gums

Clean, healthy teeth and gums will make you look good and feel more self-confident. In addition to regular visits to the dentist at least once or twice a year, you should:

- brush your teeth and gums two or three times a day after meals, using a fluoride toothpaste, to remove the debris between the teeth and gums where plaque forms
- use dental floss or tape and toothpicks with care to avoid damaging the gums
- consider using stimulator tips made of rubber to improve the circulation through the gums
- cut down on sugary foods
- eat cheese at the end of a meal to neutralise mouth acids
- ask your dentist about fluoride supplements.

D-i-y health checks

Regular self-examination of your testicles, skin and mouth is an essential part of helping yourself to stay physically healthy. You are the person most familiar with your body and its appearance, shape and feel and are therefore in the best position to notice the early-warning signs of diseases such as cancer.

Examining your testicles

All men should get into the habit of regularly examining their testicles for the appearance of lumps or irregularities, or a change in their size, shape or firmness, in the same way that women are encouraged to examine their breasts. Although cancer of the testicle is relatively rare compared with other types of cancer, it is still the most common cancer in young men aged between 20 and 35. If detected early, it is one of the easiest to cure.

Self-examination of the testicles is best performed after a warm bath or shower, when the scrotal skin is loose and relaxed. Support the scrotum and testicles in the palm of the hand to check their weight and size. Using both hands, gently roll each testicle in turn between the thumb and index and middle fingers. Any change in either testicle should be reported to your doctor as soon as possible.

Examining your skin

A regular skin check is important, not only to detect cancer but also to identify any change that might indicate some other health problem. As with testicular cancer, the sooner skin cancer is discovered and treated, the better the chance of achieving a complete cure.

Skin self-examination is particularly important for those men who have a greater risk of skin cancer, perhaps because they have:

- a fair complexion
- been regularly exposed to strong sunlight without covering up
- a large number of moles
- moles which are large, irregular in shape and patchy in colour
- a previous skin cancer
- a close relative who has had skin cancer.

Warning signs to look out for during a skin check include a change in skin texture or colour, a mole or blemish that changes in shape, size or colour, or that starts to itch or bleed, a sore or ulcer that fails to heal within three weeks and the sudden appearance of a new mole.

Checking inside your mouth

In addition to regular appointments with your dentist, it is a good idea to examine the inside of your own mouth regularly using a mirror. This is particularly important for men who smoke or drink heavily, as they are more likely to develop a mouth cancer. Changes in the mouth to look out for and report to your dentist or doctor include:

- recurrent mouth or gum bleeding
- the appearance of a new lump or swelling
- a persistent white patch, which may be a pre-cancerous condition (leukoplakia)
- any sore area on the lip, gum or inside of the mouth that fails to heal within three weeks
- numbness or pain inside the mouth for no apparent reason.

Cancer warning symptoms

As many as one in three men will develop cancer at some time in their lives. It is therefore important to be alert to the various early-warning symptoms of cancer. The point is not to become a neurotic hypochondriac, totally obsessed with the idea that any vague symptom you might develop is almost certainly the result of cancer, but to know which specific symptoms to have checked out by your doctor.

The actual cause of one of these symptoms is often something much less serious. However, ruling out cancer will put your mind at rest and in those few cases where cancer is confirmed, treatment can be started before too much damage is done and before the cancer has advanced to a stage where it can no longer be dealt with successfully. Some cancer early-warning symptoms to be aware of are:

- coughing up blood
- hoarseness that recurs or persists for longer than one week
- unexplained lumps or bumps
- swallowing difficulty that persists
- abdominal pain that recurs or persists
- unexplained constipation or diarrhoea that is prolonged for more than a week
- rectal bleeding, particularly when blood is mixed with faeces

- blood in urine
- unexplained weight loss
- headaches that persist or recur
- change in shape, size or firmness of a testicle
- bruising without injury
- a mole that changes shape, size or colour, bleeds or itches
- a scab, sore or ulcer that fails to heal within three weeks
- a persistent white patch inside the mouth.

Routine check-ups

Eye tests

Even though it is now possible to test your own eyes in some pharmacies and supermarkets to see whether you need reading glasses and what strength of lenses to choose, these d-i-y eye tests are not a substitute for a proper check-up with a professional optician because they are unable to detect other disorders that affect the eye.

You should have your eyes tested at least every two years, particularly over the age of 40, as a slow deterioration in your eyesight will often develop unnoticed. Full eye tests also allow potentially serious, sight-threatening conditions such as glaucoma (*see pages 198–9*) to be detected and treated before there is any permanent damage. A regular glaucoma test is essential for people who have a close relative (parent or brother/sister) who has suffered from this disorder, as it tends to run in families. In this situation, the eye test will be free after the age of 40. Anyone with a medical condition that can damage the blood vessels at the back of the eyes, for example, high blood pressure or diabetes, should have his vision tested at least once a year. Sudden changes in vision, such as seeing coloured haloes around lights, blurring or distortion of images, should be checked out by your doctor.

Hearing tests

Many men wrongly assume that hearing loss is an inevitable part of getting older and can't be treated. Although it is true that as you grow older your hearing mechanism becomes less sensitive to high-frequency sounds, making conversations slightly more difficult to follow, deafness should always be checked out by your doctor.

There may be a simple cause like a build-up of wax in the ear canals, or fluid behind the eardrums. Even when there is a fault in the complex hearing mechanism inside the inner ear, your doctor can arrange hearing tests at the local ear, nose and throat (ENT) clinic to determine the pattern, type and severity of the deafness and to establish whether a hearing aid would be beneficial.

Visiting the dentist

Many men avoid going to the dentist because they wrongly believe that the more they go, the more likely they are to have unnecessary treatment. Nowadays, however, most dentists are much more conservative in their approach, their main aim being to preserve the health of your teeth and gums.

Measures such as scaling and polishing can prevent the onset of tooth decay and gum disease by removing residual plaque and calculus. Dental X-rays may also be taken to reveal cavities and the spread of gum disease causing erosion of the jaw bone. These conditions can then be treated before they cause more serious damage, avoiding the need for more radical procedures.

Medical checks

A thorough medical examination may be required for a number of different reasons, for example, before starting a new job, as part of the application for a licence to drive a taxi or heavy goods vehicle, or when taking out a life assurance or personal health insurance policy.

Many men also ask their doctor for a health check because they are seeking reassurance. They may be worried about the effect of their unhealthy lifestyle but reluctant to change their habits; or someone close to them may have been taken ill or died unexpectedly.

It is dangerous, however, to regard a routine medical as a form of MOT certificate, in other words, as a clean bill of health that lasts a year. Only certain medical disorders will be picked up by even the most thorough physical examination and range of tests. And if you continue to follow an unhealthy lifestyle, you are unlikely to stay in good physical condition.

The following list of recommended screening procedures includes only those examinations and tests which can reliably diagnose a disorder at an early stage, normally before it has caused any symptoms, and where early treatment increases the chance of a cure or of preventing the development of complications.

TABLE 5

Screening test	Why done?	When recommended?
Weight	To detect excessive weight gain/loss, both of which can harm physical health	Every three years
Blood pressure (BP)	To check condition of heart and circulation	Every five years from age 20 and annually after age 50. Twice a year (at least) if on BP treatment
Urine test	To detect diabetes, kidney disease, urine infection	Every three years. With urinary symptoms, as soon as possible
Blood sugar	To diagnose diabetes	Every 5–10 years, but normally only if you are obese or have a diabetic in your close family
Blood fats (cholesterol)	Risk factor for heart and circulation disease	Every 5–10 years, but normally only if you smoke, have high blood pressure, or someone in your close family has diabetes or heart disease
Bowel screening (sigmoidoscopy and examination of faeces for blood)	To detect bowel cancer	Annual test for men over 50 (controversial). Started at an earlier age in men with ulcerative colitis or if someone in their family had bowel polyps or cancer
Prostate screening: digital rectal examination, ultrasound scan, test for blood level of prostate specific antigen	To detect prostate cancer	No clear recommendation at present

Immunisation

Immunisation is not just for children. Adults may be advised to have some or all of the following:

Influenza   Annual 'flu jabs are recommended for anyone likely to become seriously ill or to develop complications during an attack of 'flu. This includes people over the age of 65, or individuals of any age who are suffering from a chest, heart or kidney condition, or who are receiving treatment which suppresses their immune system. 'Flu jabs are also given to groups working in an institution, such as teachers and nurses, to reduce the chance of staff shortages during an epidemic.

Tetanus   A full course of three jabs is recommended for all adults who have not been vaccinated before, consisting of two doses four weeks apart and a third dose six months later. Tetanus boosters are recommended at least every ten years, with the first two boosters given routinely and any subsequent booster at the time of a deep or dirty wound, particularly one contaminated by soil, in which tetanus spores live.

Hepatitis A   This type of liver infection is on the increase; a new vaccine which gives long-term protection may be recommended for health-care workers, food handlers, sewage workers, male homosexuals and intravenous drug users.

Hepatitis B   This serious liver infection, which can cause cancer of the liver in later life, is passed on through contact with contaminated blood or other body fluids; it is far more contagious than the AIDS virus, although it may be transmitted from one person to another in similar ways.

Immunisation against hepatitis B is recommended for health-care workers, male homosexuals, intravenous drug users and family contacts or sexual partners of anyone with this infection. Police officers and prison warders are also advised to request this vaccine because of the relatively high incidence of hepatitis B among criminals, combined with the high risk of being injured at work.

Tuberculosis (TB)   The incidence of tuberculosis is on the increase again. Adults who have not received a BCG vaccination in the past should have a skin test to check their immunity (which could have developed as the result of previous exposure) before immunisation is carried out.

Polio   Assuming the recommended immunisation against polio was completed in childhood, a booster dose is needed every ten years to maintain immunity. There have been two recent cases of polio in fathers exposed to the virus as the result of contact with faeces while changing the nappy of their recently immunised babies; parents who are not immune to polio should therefore be immunised at the same time as their children.

Diphtheria   Any adult who was not immunised against diphtheria in childhood is at risk from this infection and is advised to receive a full course of three injections of low-dose vaccine one month apart.

Travel jabs   Always check with your doctor or travel agent at least two months in advance to find out which immunisations are recommended or compulsory for the countries you will be staying in or passing through. (You can obtain advice by ringing the Health Advice for Travellers★ number.)

Alcohol, smoking and drug abuse
Drinking too much

For most men, drinking alcohol is a pleasant experience and an important part of their social life. Because alcohol can help make you feel more relaxed, comfortable and sociable, it is not surprising that millions of men in the UK drink it on a regular basis.

Despite its social acceptability, however, it is important to remember that alcohol is still a drug and a highly addictive one at that. The more alcohol you drink and the more frequently you drink, the greater the risk of becoming psychologically or physically dependent on alcohol. There is a very fine dividing line between someone who drinks socially and someone who actually needs to drink every day to avoid unpleasant withdrawal symptoms.

Heavy drinkers are aware that over-indulgence can have unpleasant short-term consequences in the form of a terrible hangover the following day, but most do not realise how destructive regular alcohol abuse can be to their long-term physical health.

Drinking alcohol regularly is associated with an increased tolerance to its effects: the body adapts to the continual presence of alcohol so that you have to consume a lot more to notice any change in the way you feel. However, just because a heavy drinker no longer appears to be getting drunk doesn't mean that the large quantities of alcohol being taken in aren't causing serious damage to his body.

Alcohol in excess can be harmful to many different organs and tissues over a period of several years:

- brain – loss of memory, intellectual deterioration, depression and eventually dementia
- skin – persistent facial flushing as a result of blood-vessel damage
- heart and circulation – increased risk of high blood pressure, heart attacks and stroke
- liver – cirrhosis, hepatitis and even liver cancer
- digestive system – gastritis, pancreatitis, peptic ulcer and cancer of the mouth, throat or oesophagus
- nerves – temporary or permanent numbness, tingling and weakness
- sex organs – infertility due to sperm damage, or impotence due to hormonal changes.

WARNING SYMPTOMS OF ALCOHOL ABUSE

- drinking to relieve anxiety or to lift depression
- feeling uncomfortable on going all day without a drink
- lying or feeling guilty about your drinking
- missing work or an appointment through drinking
- drinking more when friends have had enough
- arguing or fighting under the influence of alcohol
- loss of memory, or an attack of the shakes the next day
- intense craving for a drink.

How to reduce your alcohol consumption

There are a number of ways to cut down your consumption of alcohol:

- set yourself a limit before starting and stick to it; learn to say no
- begin with a long soft drink to quench your thirst
- alternate alcoholic and non-alcoholic drinks
- have a mixer such as lemonade or tonic to dilute your drinks
- sip, do not gulp; appreciate the flavour of your drink
- aim for two alcohol-free days a week; you may need to avoid drinking partners and places on those days
- switch to alcohol-free or low-alcohol wines or beers
- keep a diary to identify when and where most of your drinking takes place.

Safe alcohol limits

Alcohol is unlikely to harm your health if you drink only small amounts and avoid drinking every day. In fact, alcohol in moderation has been shown to be good for your heart and circulation, with a protective effect against heart attacks and angina.

The risks of alcohol, described above, are associated with drinking large quantities regularly over several years. Doctors recommend that men should keep their average weekly intake of alcohol below a maximum of 21 units to avoid damaging their health.

A unit of alcohol, roughly equivalent to eight grams, represents half a pint of ordinary beer or lager, one glass of table wine, one small glass of sherry or one single pub measure of spirits. Remember, however, that some real ales and extra-strength lagers contain up to two-and-a-half times as much alcohol as ordinary beer or lager, that fortified wine such as port contains up to twice as much alcohol as ordinary wine and that when you are serving spirits at home you are probably a lot more generous than the pub when it comes to pouring a measure. Cider ranges from between one-and-a-half to two units for a half-pint depending on its strength.

Getting help for an alcohol problem

Unfortunately, most men who are abusing alcohol are either unaware that they have a problem or refuse to admit it. If you or someone close to you is drinking in excess, the first point of contact should be your family doctor or the local branch of Alcoholics Anonymous*. While it is not possible to force someone to go for treatment, it is worth trying to reason with the person at a time when he is sober. Alcoholics Anonymous offers advice and guidance for people with a drink problem and provides support to the whole family (try also ALANON*). In severe cases, it may be necessary to admit an alcoholic to hospital for a period of detoxification, with medication prescribed to control the unpleasant withdrawal symptoms.

Long-term treatment to prevent a return to previous drinking habits can include behavioural therapy and psychotherapy; occasionally, a drug known as disulfuram is prescribed, which induces unpleasant side-effects when taken with alcohol.

Smoking – more than just a cancer risk

Cigarette smoking is the most important self-inflicted cause of illness and premature death in Western countries. Smoking has been directly linked with cancers of the lung, mouth, throat, larynx, oesophagus and bladder. In addition, smokers appear to have a higher risk of cancers of the pancreas, kidney and stomach.

While most men are aware of the cancer risk from smoking, there are also many other less well-publicised smoking-related diseases. A smoker's cough may progress to chronic bronchitis and emphysema, causing breathlessness severe enough to stop someone leading a normal lifestyle. Smokers also have a much greater chance of suffering from angina, heart attacks or a stroke, or of needing an amputation because of blocked circulation in one or more of their limbs.

It is generally never too late to benefit from giving up smoking. For example, the risk of premature death from a heart attack or chronic bronchitis is almost halved within five years of quitting tobacco.

How to give up smoking
Nearly four out of every five smokers say they would like to quit, encouraged by the knowledge that they would almost certainly improve their life expectancy and their quality of life. However, the fact that only about one-quarter of those who try manage to give up demonstrates how powerfully addictive the smoking habit is. Quitline* offers advice to smokers who want to give up.

To improve your chance of quitting successfully, try to identify the reasons why you smoke. Then you can adopt the tactics best suited to the type of smoker you are.

The nicotine addict Smokers who suffer unpleasant withdrawal symptoms, such as headaches, anxiety, irritability and an intense craving for a cigarette can benefit from a nicotine substitute in the form of chewing gum or skin patches. Ask your doctor or pharmacist for advice and counselling on how best to use nicotine-replacement therapy.

Smoking to socialise This type of smoker should avoid the places where he will be tempted or encouraged to smoke and keep away from friends who will continue to offer him cigarettes.

Smoking to relieve tension Use other techniques to reduce stress, such as a new hobby, playing sport or learning a relaxation exercise (see **Chapter 3**).

Smoking to occupy hands and mouth Chew sugar-free gum to keep your mouth busy, play with worry beads to distract your fingers.

Smoking to fight boredom Become interested in a new activity, preferably one that occupies your hands, such as learning to play the guitar or model-making.

Smoking as a routine At those times you invariably light up a cigarette, after a meal, for example, do something else.

EXTRA TIPS ON GIVING UP

- make a list of all your reasons for quitting
- choose a time when you are not going to be highly stressed
- stop abruptly at a set time; cutting down gradually rarely works
- give up with a friend who can offer extra support
- throw away cigarettes, lighters, ashtrays etc.
- avoid chocolate, red meat, tea, coffee and alcohol, which can all increase craving
- drink plenty of water, fruit juice and herbal tea
- spend the money you save on cigarettes on something special
- consider hypnosis or acupuncture if you are having difficulty stopping.

THE WHICH? GUIDE TO MEN'S HEALTH

Weight gain

Some men find that they put on a few kilograms in weight after they give up smoking. This is partly because they are no longer taking in nicotine, which stimulates the body's metabolism, and partly because their appetite will tend to increase as a result of better awareness of taste. However, if you only nibble on healthy snacks (*see page 61*), you are unlikely to put on more than a few kilograms, and being a little overweight is nowhere near as bad for your health as continuing to smoke.

Drug abuse – the risks

A wide variety of drugs may be misused, including some drugs normally prescribed by a doctor, such as painrelievers, stimulants, tranquillisers and anabolic steroids. In such cases, they are often taken in amounts far in excess of the normal dosage. Other drugs that are commonly misused, such as cannabis, Ecstasy, LSD, amphetamine, cocaine and crack cocaine, are either home-grown, manufactured illicitly in home laboratories, or illegally imported from abroad.

There are many different reasons for abusing drugs, including the desire to escape from reality, the search for self-awareness, trying to achieve a mystical experience, or simply a curiosity about the effects. Amphetamines and anabolic steroids are sometimes abused in an attempt to improve sporting performance.

Regular or excessive use of a drug may lead to addiction, either in the form of psychological dependence, in which the individual experiences severe emotional distress or intense craving when that drug is no longer being taken, or physical dependence, in which stopping the drug abruptly results in unpleasant withdrawal symptoms that may last several days.

Tolerance to a drug may also develop with regular usage, which will make it necessary to use progressively larger amounts of the drug to achieve the same effect. Drug dependence almost inevitably leads to a deterioration in physical as well as emotional health, in addition to the financial problems related to paying for the habit and probably becoming unfit for work.

Tranquillisers (e.g. benzodiazepines) Nowadays, doctors generally prescribe these drugs only for short periods in as low a dosage as possible. Regular use for more than two weeks is likely to lead to physical dependence. After long-term prescription, the dose of benzodiazepine has to be reduced gradually over several weeks to avoid unpleasant withdrawal symptoms. Due to their calming, relaxing effect, benzodiazepines are commonly abused, particularly by people abusing other drugs, such as opiates and stimulants.

Barbiturates   These sedative drugs are still prescribed for epilepsy and occasionally for insomnia. Like benzodiazepines, a barbiturate may be abused for its relaxing, calming effect. Regular use leads to physical dependence and accidental overdose can be fatal if it stops the normal breathing mechanism.

Opiate drugs   These narcotic painrelievers, which include heroin, morphine and dihydrocodeine, are used medically to treat severe pain. They are abused because of their ability to induce a state of euphoria. Regular misuse of an opiate leads to physical dependence and accidental overdose can cause coma and death if the breathing mechanism is suppressed.

Amphetamines   These stimulant drugs, which were once commonly prescribed as appetite suppressants, are abused to induce feelings of excitement and boost energy levels, particularly by individuals who are suffering the effects of fatigue or lack of sleep. Regular amphetamine abuse can result in paranoia or aggressive behaviour. An overdose may cause palpitations, hallucinations, a dangerous rise in blood pressure and, on rare occasions, seizures.

Ecstasy ('E')   This powerful stimulant, chemically similar to amphetamine, has become popular among young people. Although many have taken this drug with no apparent ill effects, there have been several deaths and a number of serious adverse psychiatric and physical reactions as a result of the action of this drug on the brain, heart, muscles and other parts of the body. When Ecstasy is used at parties or 'raves' the chance of heat exhaustion and dehydration may be reduced by wearing loose cotton clothing and drinking copious amounts of non-alcoholic fluids.

Potentially fatal toxic effects have included seizures, hepatitis, kidney failure and a dangerous increase in body temperature. Risks are greater when large numbers of Ecstasy tablets are taken at once or if the tablets have been adulterated with other drugs, such as amphetamine and LSD, or other harmful substances.

LSD This powerful hallucinogenic drug, which was once used in psychiatric patients receiving psychotherapy, produces unpredictable effects with bizarre hallucinations that may be pleasant or terrifying. Several people have died while under the influence of LSD, for example, by trying to fly from an upper floor window and, occasionally, a single dose leads to prolonged psychosis in a vulnerable individual.

Cocaine This drug, originally obtained from the leaves of plants growing naturally in South America, is now also produced synthetically. Its rapid action on the skin and mucous membrane surfaces, which lasts for up to an hour, made cocaine an ideal anaesthetic for minor surgical procedures involving the eye, ear, nose or throat. Because it also narrows the blood vessels, its anaesthetic effect remains localised.

Absorbed into the main bloodstream, however, cocaine interferes with normal brain chemistry to induce feelings of increased energy, well-being, elation and euphoria. This has led to widespread abuse of cocaine, usually by inhalation through the nose (snorting). As a result of this abuse potential, doctors have switched to using other types of local anaesthetic.

Regular snorting of cocaine powder can damage the lining of the nose, causing uncomfortable congestion in the short term and, eventually, total tissue destruction, with perforation of the nasal septum. People who regularly abuse cocaine are likely to become psychologically dependent on it, experiencing intense cravings for the next high. Large doses may cause a psychotic reaction, seizures or cardiac arrest.

Crack cocaine Crack is a purified form of cocaine made by a process known as free-basing to produce small rocks about the size of raisins. Smoking crack induces a much more intense and rapid psychological effect than sniffing cocaine powder, with extreme euphoria and a sense of heightened physical and mental capacity. However, these feelings wear off within about 12 minutes leaving the user severely anxious or depressed, with loss of appetite and difficulty in sleeping. Frequent doses are therefore required to sustain a high. Regular crack smoking may cause a chronic cough, wheeze and a partial loss of voice. Long-standing abuse also leads to suicidal feelings, unpredictable behaviour, delusions and hallucinations. As with cocaine powder, a crack overdose can result in seizures and cardiac arrest.

Marijuana   This popular recreational drug comes from the flowering tops and dried leaves of the Indian hemp plant *Cannabis sativa*. It is used for its ability to cause euphoria, enhanced perception, feelings of relaxation and pleasant drowsiness, with time seeming to pass more slowly. The lack of physical and psychological problems associated with marijuana has led to a campaign to legalise it. However, it may aggravate or unmask a psychiatric condition in someone who was already at risk and is known to impair short-term memory.

Giving up marijuana after regular use does not produce unpleasant withdrawal symptoms, but persistent use may cause apathy or depression. There is a concern about the influence marijuana may have on driving, due to its effect on visuo-spatial judgement, but this has not been supported by accident statistics.

Individuals who smoke marijuana with tobacco, rather than on its own, are exposed to all the health risks associated with cigarette smoking (*see page 92*).

Solvents   More than 100 domestic products, including glue and cleaning fluid, may be deliberately inhaled to induce euphoria or hallucinations. Continued inhalation can rapidly lead to drowsiness, loss of co-ordination, slurred speech and disorientation. Severe intoxication occasionally results in seizures, coma and death. Other risks include asphyxia during inhalation and accidents occurring while under the influence of the solvent. Long-term toxic effects from regular solvent abuse include brain, liver and kidney damage.

Anabolic steroids   These drugs regularly hit the headlines when an athlete or sportsperson is found to have traces of anabolic steroid in his or her urine. The reason for abusing this type of drug is to boost the development of strong, bulky muscles. By speeding up the recovery of muscles after a strenuous workout in the gym, anabolic steroids allow a more demanding training programme. Each of the authorities governing the various competitive sports has banned the use of anabolic steroids, not only because they confer an unfair advantage, but also due to their potential to cause serious side-effects, such as liver damage and infertility.

Overcoming drug addiction

If you or someone close to you has become dependent on any drug, the first step is to seek professional help through, for example, your family doctor or by contacting an organisation such as Release★ or the Standing Conference on Drug Abuse (SCODA)★. The addict will usually be referred to a specialised drug rehabilitation centre, where a gradual withdrawal from the substance can be followed through under careful medical supervision.

Once a drug habit has been overcome, professional counselling, psychotherapy or behaviour therapy may be recommended to help prevent a relapse. Self-help groups can assist motivation to stay off drugs; it is also crucial to break with drug-taking friends, to move to new surroundings and to form new relationships.

CHAPTER 3

COPING WITH STRESS

MANY men thrive on stress; they are unhappy unless there are dead-lines to meet and more than one job on the go at any one time. A performer on stage or an athlete in competition will often find the inherant stress exhilarating. The way in which you handle stress is determined partly by your personality and partly by your innate ability to cope under different types of pressure. However, there is also a great deal you can do to enable stress to work for you, rather than work against you.

Stress under control can be a positive force that improves perfor-mance, provides stimulation and motivation and keeps you on your toes and out of danger. Some degree of stress is essential to add spice to your life and prevent you from becoming bored and apathetic.

All men experience intense stress at certain times in their life, for example, when circumstances suddenly change or an event beyond their control occurs. However, stress overload increases the risk of both mental and physical illnesses, as well as increasing susceptibility to accidental injuries. Over half of all visits to the doctor are thought to be related in some way to stress, usually in the form of worries about work or money.

Causes of stress

Stress is triggered by an activity or circumstance that arouses the emotions or is perceived to be a threat or danger. This includes a wide variety of stimuli: for example, being on the receiving end of verbal or physical aggression; a traumatic life event such as losing your job or moving house; or an internal conflict, such as guilt.

All these stressful situations cause characteristic physical changes in the body, which represent a primitive reaction to stress that enabled our ancestors either to fight or to escape from everyday dangers ('fight or flight'). This response occurs as a result of the release of stress hormones – adrenaline, noradrenaline and cortisol – from the activated adrenal glands and stimulation of the sympathetic nerves around the body. Physical changes brought on by stress prepare the body to perform to maximum efficiency:

● heart beats stronger and more rapidly
● breathing becomes deeper and faster
● muscles receive greater blood flow
● sweating increases to prevent overheating
● pupils widen to let in more light; eyes focus for distance vision
● blood sugar levels rise to provide an energy source for muscles.

Harmful effects of stress

Ideally, stress is a temporary condition that arises to meet a specific challenge and subsides once those demands have been resolved. After a short period of stress, the body is then allowed to return to its resting state. Problems arise when:

● the threat is mental or emotional rather than physical, in which case the 'fight or flight' response is unhelpful. Changes, such as a more rapid heartbeat, increased muscle tension and sweating, do not provide a defence against psychological pressure and there is no opportunity to work off your arousal through physical exertion
● the threat is prolonged, for example, constant pressure from a demanding job or an unhappy relationship. People who are unable to escape from or conquer their source of stress remain in a heightened state of arousal and the result of this continuous and unwanted tension is likely to be an adverse effect on both mental and physical health.

Stressful life events

Some people find even relatively minor irritations like a queue at a ticket office or being held up in a traffic jam stressful, while others are able to stay calm and relaxed. There are, however, a number of traumatic life events that cause great stress for almost everyone: for example, the death of your partner, being sent to jail, divorce, losing your job, impending fatherhood.

Although a particular change in his life may cause more stress for one man than for another, it is still possible to predict the risk of stress-related illness from the number and nature of life events which an individual has been through.

Warning symptoms

Many men are unaware of just how much stress they are under. They fail to recognise the early-warning symptoms of stress overload. It is only when you acknowledge the harmful levels of stress in your life that you will be able to do something positive to protect your emotional and physical health.

Common symptoms of stress include:

- difficulty falling asleep
- inability to concentrate or make decisions
- increasing irritability, impatience and loss of temper
- constantly feeling tired or lethargic
- eating when not hungry
- smoking more, drinking more alcohol
- recurrent headaches, muscle or joint pains
- reduced interest in sex
- driving fast and dangerously.

Stress-related illness

Almost every illness has some link with your state of mind and your emotions; feeling depressed can make a physical condition seem a lot more serious than it really is. The term 'psychosomatic' is used to describe any illness that appears to have been caused or aggravated by psychological factors. This does not mean that a psychosomatic illness is imaginary, simply that emotional problems are a major influence on the condition. Common disorders that are sometimes, but not always, psychosomatic include irritable bowel syndrome and tension headaches. Anyone who has suffered from these conditions will know just how genuine the symptoms are.

Prolonged minor stresses or a source of intense stress may contribute to a variety of disorders affecting different parts of the body:

- skin – eczema and psoriasis may both flare up during times of stress
- reproductive organs – stress is the most common cause of impotence and premature ejaculation
- digestive system – stress-related problems include gastritis, peptic ulcer, irritable bowel and colitis
- immune system – stress is known to increase susceptibility to infection
- heart and circulation – stress can increase blood pressure, which in turn raises the risk of suffering a heart attack
- lungs – emotional upset may aggravate some cases of asthma
- hair – baldness is occasionally brought on by extreme stress
- brain – stress may be the cause of many mental and emotional problems, such as anxiety and depression. The popular term 'nervous breakdown' refers to a stress-related condition in which the individual is no longer able to deal with everyday problems.

Coping with stress

While it is clearly impossible, as well as undesirable, to avoid stress altogether, there is a lot you can do to improve your ability to cope with stressful situations and prevent stress overload. First, you need to recognise the early-warning symptoms of stress, as described above. Then you should attempt to identify the various sources of stress in your life and decide what you are going to do about them. Any action you take to relieve stress is bound to do some good because it is an indication that you are no longer prepared to put up with this unacceptable level of pressure.

If you are having trouble pinpointing the exact cause of your stress, make a note of the circumstances each time you start to feel more anxious and see whether a pattern emerges. The key to reducing stress is to deal with one problem at a time. Make a list, in order of priority, and start with the situation that is causing the most distress, leaving the minor irritations to last.

Talk frankly to anyone you see as being at the root of your troubles. Admitting that things are getting on top of you may be an awkward or embarrassing confession to make to your partner, your children, your parents or your boss. The sooner you involve the other person, however, the sooner you will be able to find a constructive solution.

It is also important to express your emotions openly, rather than trying to bottle them up. Don't be afraid to show that you are angry or sad; crying doesn't reflect a loss of masculinity, nor does it mean you will lose the respect of those around you.

There are other ways to keep your stress levels under control:

- where possible, avoid making too many changes in your life at once
- don't brood about situations or events over which you have no control
- don't feel guilty about having to change arrangements or ideas
- cultivate your social life – all work and no play damages health
- exercise regularly to release pent-up emotions, reduce tension, take your mind off any particular worries and encourage deep, refreshing sleep
- use a regular relaxation technique, such as breathing exercises, muscle relaxation, meditation, yoga or massage.

If you are unable to sort out your stress-related problems on your own using the self-help measures and relaxation techniques described in this chapter, do not delay going to see your doctor, particularly if you feel the stress in your life is out of control, making you feel ill, or preventing you from leading a normal life. You may need counselling to help you adjust your outlook or lifestyle. If your case is severe, you may need medication to lift your depression or suppress your anxiety.

Managing stress at home

Stress in the home is often more intense than many people realise, with a wide variety of potential problems straining the emotional health of each family member. The father, for example, may be put under increased stress by the arrival of a new baby, his daughter leaving home, his wife going back to work, the death of one of his parents. His response to these events and the way the rest of the family responds add up to a complex mix of stresses. Different families will be affected in different ways, and some will handle the situation a lot better than others.

The best way to cope during and after any period of domestic stress is to allow everyone in the family to communicate their feelings and fears as far as possible. It is also essential to try to appreciate the stress other family members are under.

Remember that the person who stays at home to look after the children is not taking the easy option. Running a home and raising children is a full-time occupation which is usually highly stressful; many women do this and a paid job as well.

Many parents do not realise just how much stress their children are putting them under and wrongly feel guilty if they lose patience with them. A child may continually demand attention and, if one or both parents' sleep is being regularly disturbed, he or she is likely to end up exhausted and irritable. Ways to cope with this type of stress are discussed in detail in **Chapter 5**.

If money worries are a major factor behind the build-up of stress in your home, contact your bank or a financial adviser for help. Don't make the mistake of just ignoring all the people you owe money to – banks and building societies are much more sympathetic if you explain your situation, and can help you organise a system of repayment.

When someone in the family is violent or has an alcohol or drug problem, the resultant pressures in the home will put all the family members at risk of stress-related illness. In this situation it is vital to seek professional help, starting with your GP or the Samaritans★.

Marriage breakdown

One in three marriages in the UK ends in divorce and second marriages are even less likely to work. Warning symptoms that your relationship with your partner is under threat include:

- difficulty talking about personal problems
- frequent arguments or fits of temper which you then regret
- intense jealousy
- believing you are contributing a lot more than your partner
- feeling trapped or held back
- no longer looking forward to coming home
- an unsatisfying sex life with your partner
- a desire for other sexual relationships.

Holidays are a common time for relationship difficulties to come to the surface. Couples wrongly expect everything to be fine away from the pressures of work; but, in reality, the holiday takes them away from the activities they were using to avoid each other and forces them to confront their conflicting attitudes and emotions.

Saving your relationship

Married couples or established partners who are going through a bad patch in their relationship, which they have been unable to sort out themselves, often benefit from professional counselling. For some couples, however, divorce or separation provides a welcome release from the stress of living with an incompatible partner.

You can make an appointment with one of the counsellors employed by the national organisation Relate★ (formerly the Marriage Guidance Council). Alternatively, you can see your GP, who may be trained in counselling, or you may be referred to a clinical psychologist who specialises in marital problems.

Partners should attend the counselling sessions together on a regular basis. Marital therapy begins with an analysis of the good and bad aspects of the relationship, with both parties encouraged to express openly their grievances and how they would like to see an improvement. Any blame for the marriage/relationship problems should be shared equally.

In addition to learning to communicate more effectively with each other, couples should try to find a leisure activity that they can both enjoy together. Sex therapy may also be recommended, although any problems with a sexual relationship will only be resolved once difficulties outside the bedroom have been overcome.

Stress management at work

If you feel under stress as a result of your job, try to identify which of the following reasons apply to your situation at work:

- no control over your workload
- recently passed over for promotion
- threat of redundancy
- too much/not enough responsibility
- working long hours

- having to take work home
- excessive competition
- hostility from colleagues
- sexual harassment (*see opposite*)
- unrealistic deadlines
- no procedure to settle grievances
- enforced relocation to a new area
- boredom
- job dissatisfaction
- working only for the money
- difficult or uncomfortable journey to and from work
- demotion
- unwanted promotion
- conflict of loyalties
- unpleasant confrontation with the public.

If nothing is done to resolve your problems at work you are likely to become ill. The symptoms may be back pain or depression, but the real reason is job-related stress.

Changing your approach

Many men could regain control of the stress related to their work by managing their time more effectively and taking regular time out to relax and unwind. To improve your time-management skills, stick to the following principles – you will soon notice an improvement both in your productivity and the way you feel about your job.

- It is important not to waste time procrastinating. Prepare a list of the tasks you need to accomplish in order of priority. Set yourself realistic goals and say no to unreasonable demands and impracticable deadlines. Finish one job before you move on to the next.
- Divide large projects into more manageable chunks and delegate work to others when you can.
- Take regular breaks during the day. A brief rest period will help refresh your mind after a long session of concentrated mental effort and stop you becoming frustrated with a project. It is best to go for a change in scenery, for example, by taking a walk in a nearby park, if possible.
- Transfer any uncompleted task to the following day's action plan and make a note of anything that interfered with your work

schedule which you may be able to rectify; it may be necessary, for example, to have someone take phone messages for part of the day to avoid constant interruptions.

- Take weekend breaks and proper holidays, preferably away from home, to prevent you getting stuck into potentially stressful activities like clearing out the garage.

Clearly some of the problems listed at the beginning of this section cannot be solved simply by changing your approach to work. Ideally, you should communicate your difficulties either directly to your boss or indirectly via your union or staff committee. However, you should be aware of the need to handle the situation tactfully to avoid being seen as a troublemaker.

If you decide to try your hand at something different, think about gaining extra qualifications in your spare time before putting in your notice. Men stuck in a bad job situation should concentrate on achieving fulfilment and enjoyment from their life outside of work.

SEXUAL HARASSMENT

It is not just women who get sexually harassed; men may be harassed by women or other men at work.

If this is happening to you, try to avoid contact with the individual as far as possible, although this may be difficult within the confines of an office or shop floor. Be assertive by making it clear that you find this behaviour offensive, but there is no need to be rude.

If the situation doesn't improve, you will need to make a formal complaint. In the meantime, keep a detailed diary of each episode of harassment and the circumstances in which it occurred as this will help you prepare your case. Also, discreetly ask your male colleagues whether they have been experiencing the same problem.

Relaxation techniques

Relaxation is a skill that everyone should learn because it is an essential part of a healthy lifestyle. It doesn't matter which of the many techniques you choose to help you relax, but you should practise regularly to gain the maximum benefit for your physical and emotional health. Regular use of a relaxation technique will also make it easier for you to cope during periods of more intense stress. In addition to reducing muscle tension, daily relaxation will help relieve stress-related conditions, such as recurrent headaches and back pain.

Breathing exercise

Try the following exercise for five minutes at a time twice a day and then use it whenever you start to feel tense or anxious:

- find a quiet area where you won't be disturbed by people or the telephone
- sit in a comfortable chair with your feet flat on the floor, relax your shoulders and become aware of the chair supporting you
- consciously slow your rate of breathing and take deep, even breaths
- breathe out for twice as long as you breathe in, controlling this pattern by silently counting to yourself
- during this breathing exercise, try to clear your mind of all thoughts and worries
- stop deep breathing if you begin to feel dizzy.

Muscle relaxation

Muscles that have become tense and taut can be relaxed by the following simple routine. Find somewhere that is quiet, warm and dimly lit where you won't be disturbed; take off your shoes and remove any spectacles or contact lenses before you begin. Ideally, you should be wearing comfortable, loose-fitting clothing which allows you to move each part of your body freely.

- lie flat on your back either on a bed or the floor
- close your eyes, let all your muscles go limp and breathe at your normal resting rate and rhythm
- tighten the muscles in your toes for a few seconds before relaxing them as you breathe out
- work up your body, tightening and then relaxing each group of muscles in turn
- when you reach your face, screw up the muscles around your mouth and eyes, then let them relax as if the skin on your face is sliding off on to the floor
- raise your head for a few seconds, then relax your neck and jaw

muscles to allow your head to fall gently back and your mouth and throat to open

- repeat this whole toe-to-head sequence until ten minutes have passed, then lie completely still for a few more minutes; you should feel totally relaxed
- stretch your arms and legs gently before going back into action.

Meditation

Traditionally, meditation has been an integral part of many different religions, particularly those based on Eastern philosophies. People experienced in meditation often use these techniques as a pathway towards spiritual awareness and fulfilment. For most people in the West, however, the aim of meditation is simply to release inner tension and achieve a state of deep relaxation by emptying the mind of distracting thoughts and worries.

A variety of organisations teach meditation. The most common form practised in the West is transcendental meditation (TM)(★), in which the individual is given a personal secret word or sound (a *mantra*) by the instructor to say over and over again to himself.

To see if meditation works for you, try the following simple exercise. Find a quiet room where you won't be disturbed and try to sit cross-legged with your back straight, but modify this position as necessary to get comfortable. Breathe at your normal resting rate and rhythm, close your eyes and choose one of these techniques to empty your mind of thoughts and ideas:

- repeat a word or phrase silently to yourself without moving your lips; the word or words should have no emotional significance so you can concentrate on the exercise itself and not think about the meaning
- imagine a beautiful scene and savour every minute detail of this picture in your mind's eye
- alternatively, with your eyes open, stare at one specific stationary object such as the pattern on a wall, but don't attempt to analyse its form or shape.

Meditate for only five minutes at a time until you find it easier to clear your mind of distractions. With practice, you will gradually be able to increase your session of meditation up to a maximum of 20 minutes.

Whichever technique you follow, you will find that your mind wanders, or distracting thoughts start to intrude. The trick is to take yourself gently back to concentrating on your word, phrase, image or object each time this happens. There is no need to actively force out these distractions, simply try not to follow them and not to worry about how well you are doing.

Yoga

Although yoga is based on an ancient system of Indian philosophy and physical discipline, this activity has become increasingly popular in the West in recent decades. Not only is yoga a useful relaxation technique that helps calm the mind and reduce tension, some exercises produce physical benefits, including helping to improve flexibility, balance and co-ordination, and increasing muscle strength and endurance.

It is best to learn yoga in a supervised class. In Hatha yoga you will be taught co-ordinated movements and postures, called *asanas*, that exercise virtually every part of your body, combined with breath-control techniques known as *pranayamas*. In Siddha yoga the emphasis is on meditation techniques.

People who experiment with Hatha yoga on their own run the risk of over-stretching injuries. Elderly people and anyone with a specific medical disorder such as high blood pressure, back trouble or glaucoma (raised pressure in the eye – *see page 198*) may have to avoid or modify certain positions. (The Yoga for Health Foundation★ and the British Wheel of Yoga★ can offer advice.)

Massage

Thanks to the sex industry, massage has acquired a somewhat sleazy reputation. However, there are many *bona fide* massage practitioners who are experienced in massage techniques that have nothing to do with sexual stimulation. There are also several good books available which will teach you how to massage your partner and yourself.

Massage involves stroking, kneading and pummelling the muscles and other soft tissues in various parts of the body. It is a powerful relaxation technique which is tremendously comforting, producing a positive feeling of well-being in both the recipient and the person giving the massage. A foot massage not only makes your feet feel good but also refreshes and relaxes your whole body. A facial massage can relieve tension headaches and stress-related fatigue, as well as leaving your face looking and feeling fresher and younger.

Massage is available only in a few GPs' surgeries and hospital clinics, so most people will have to go for private treatment. Because anyone can set themselves up as a massage practitioner, without any experience or qualifications, it is advisable to visit only a chartered physiotherapist (with the letters MCSP) who offers massage therapy or someone approved by the British Massage Therapy Council*. This organisation will provide a list of practitioners in your area in return for an s.a.e.

MASSAGE SAFETY TIPS

Do not eat or drink immediately before a massage. Tense muscles may feel uncomfortable during a massage, but you should not feel sore afterwards.

Massage is not recommended for those with any of the following conditions:

- a fever or infection, including skin infection
- skin inflammation in the area to be massaged
- pain made worse or spread to other areas when pressure is applied
- thrombosis, phlebitis or varicose veins (may be aggravated by massage of the affected area).

Teach yourself massage

There is no substitute for practical tuition in the art of massage. However, here are some basic tips to get you started:

- choose a warm, dimly lit, quiet room where you won't be disturbed
- remove anything that might scratch, irritate or be distracting, such as a watch or bracelet; rings should be removed or covered with tape
- only the area being massaged should be exposed: cover the rest of the body with towels
- assuming you do not have a specialised massage couch, the person being massaged should lie on a firm padded surface, most likely a bed. If the bed does not have a firm mattress, use blankets, foam

rubber or a mattress on the floor; the masseur or masseuse should kneel on something comfortable

- to enable your hands to glide smoothly over the skin, use a light vegetable oil or talcum powder. A range of aromatherapy massage oils is available, each of which is recommended for specific disorders
- if you use a massage oil, never pour it directly on to the skin of the person being massaged. Put less than one teaspoonful into the palm of your hand and warm the oil up by rubbing your hands together
- start with circular stroking movements, moulding your hands to the contours of the body and keeping to a constant rhythm
- keep one hand in contact with the body at all times. If you need more oil, pour a little on to the back of the massaging hand and continue stroking while you use your free hand to transfer this extra oil lightly on to the skin
- during the massage, concentrate on your hand movements and don't talk too much
- on small areas, stroke with your thumbs or fingertips
- over larger muscles, use firmer pressure but don't push too hard
- if massage is causing a ticklish sensation, increase the pressure or move to a different area
- to release muscle tension, apply deep pressure with your thumbs either kept still or moving in tiny circles
- to relax tense muscles in the fleshy areas around the shoulders, hips and thighs, try a kneading technique. Pummelling with loosely clenched fists with your wrists relaxed will create a light, bouncy pressure on the muscles, which will also help.

CHAPTER 4

SEXUAL HEALTH AND AWARENESS

WHATEVER your sexual orientation, it is important to understand the principles of safer sex and to know about the symptoms and treatment of different sexually transmitted diseases. Also, because sexual arousal and responses are broadly similar in heterosexual and homosexual men, the advice given in this chapter on how to overcome relatively common psychosexual problems, such as impotence and premature ejaculation, is relevant to all men.

No attempt is made here to offer recommendations on how to vary or improve your sex life, a matter beyond the bounds of 'health', but those who want this information will find the subject amply covered in other books and in magazines and educational videos.

Safer sex

Safe sex used to mean taking precautions to avoid an unwanted pregnancy. Nowadays, with the spread of HIV (Human Immunodeficiency Virus) infection and AIDS (Acquired Immune Deficiency Syndrome), this term more commonly refers to precautions taken to protect against sexually transmitted diseases (STDs). However, because absolute protection is impossible, it is more accurate to refer to the practice of *safer* sex.

Despite all the publicity warning of the risk of HIV infection, many heterosexual men – particularly those in their 20s and 30s – do not practise safer sex. One reason for this is that some people still believe that it is only homosexual men and drug addicts who are likely to expose themselves to HIV and AIDS. In 1992, however, there were

286 new cases of HIV infection and 107 new AIDS cases among heterosexual men in the UK. Another common problem is that while many men agree that using a condom is a good idea, most don't bother in practice. They may carry condoms, but unless their partners insist that they use them, they invariably don't. A survey by the Health Education Authority revealed that only 30 per cent of 18–24-year-old men had used a condom the last time they had sex.

Even more alarming is the fact that the men least likely to use a condom are those who have the most sexual encounters and who therefore run the greatest risk of picking up and passing on sexually transmitted diseases.

SAFER SEX RECOMMENDATIONS

- When having intercourse (vaginal or anal), you should always use a condom for at least the first three months of a mutually monogamous relationship (anal sex is actually illegal in England, Wales and Northern Ireland between a man and a woman).
- Before stopping the use of condoms, you and your partner should both have a sexual health check-up at your GP's surgery or an STD clinic (*see below*).
- If both you and your partner are clear of disease and monogamous, there is no need to use a condom, except as a method of contraception (if the relationship is not mutually monogamous, condoms are still required).
- Some STDs can be passed on by oral or anal sex.

STD clinics

If you have symptoms of an STD, or have been with someone suspected or known to have an STD, it is important for you to have a check-up as soon as possible. For most types of STD, the earlier treatment is started, the less likely it is that complications will develop.

However, the STD clinic is not just for people worried about infection; clinic staff can also provide advice about sexual health and encourage both men and women to go for regular check-ups, even if they have no symptoms. A good time for a check-up is before starting a new sexual relationship, or before giving up using condoms with a regular partner.

STD clinics are listed in the telephone directory under STD, VD or genito-urinary medicine. Alternatively, the local hospital will have a GU or 'special' clinic, which you can call to make an appointment; it is not necessary to be referred by a GP. Some clinics will give you a time for an appointment over the phone, others see patients in the order they arrive. Appointments and treatment at an NHS clinic are free, private STD clinics may charge anything from £30 upwards.

You may give a false name if you prefer, but your details are completely confidential and will not be revealed to your doctor, employer, insurance company or partner without your permission. STD clinics do provide the Department of Health with information about the number of cases of a particular STD, to keep statistics up to date, but this does not include patient names or any personal details.

Whatever condition you suspect you are suffering from, it is routine practice to screen for all STDs apart from HIV, which is usually tested for only on request and with counselling about the significance of the result. After questions about your sexual habits and any symptoms you might have, your physical examination will normally include a swab being taken from the opening to the urethra at the tip of the penis; urine and blood samples will also be taken.

Some results will be available within a few minutes, but for other tests you need to telephone later or call back in person. It is usually possible for the clinic doctor to make at least a provisional diagnosis and any treatment necessary can be provided straight away.

Although not obliged to let previous or current sexual partners know about any STD you have picked up, the clinic staff will encourage you to give permission for them to get in touch with your sexual contacts. They do not have to give your name to these people; they simply advise them to attend their local clinic for treatment.

Common sexually transmitted diseases

At the beginning of this century the most common STDs were gonorrhoea and syphilis; now it is non-specific urethritis (NSU) that tops the list, along with genital warts and genital herpes. Media attention is focused mainly on HIV and AIDS, but at present the number of known cases of these conditions in the UK is relatively small compared to those of other STDs.

Non-specific urethritis (NSU)

Urethritis is inflammation of the urethra, the narrow tube that runs through the penis carrying either urine from the bladder or semen on ejaculation. The most common cause of urethritis in men, non-specific urethritis (NSU), is due to infection with chlamydia, a type of bug that has some of the characteristics of bacteria and other features that are more typical of viruses.

NSU causes a burning discomfort on passing urine and a yellowish discharge from the penis. The diagnosis may be confirmed by examining a swab of the discharge under a microscope. Treatment is with a course of antibiotics, usually a type of tetracycline. Left untreated, NSU in men may spread to infect the testicle and epididymis, causing pain, tenderness and swelling. Joint and eye inflammation are other possible complications.

All sexual partners of an NSU sufferer should also be treated with antibiotics, regardless of whether they have noticed any urethral discomfort or discharge. This is because many women who pick up a chlamydia infection remain free of urinary symptoms, or the urethral discharge is masked by their normal vaginal discharge. Men can develop inflammation of the rectum as a complication of NSU, although it may not cause any symptoms.

Gonorrhoea

Symptoms of gonorrhoea may appear at any time between two and ten days after exposure to this bacterial infection, with a discharge of pus from the urethra and pain on passing urine that can vary from a mild discomfort to a severe burning sensation. Oral sex with someone who is infected with gonorrhoea can lead to painful inflammation of the throat. Gonorrhoea picked up by anal sex can result in anal irritation and discharge due to inflammation of the rectum.

Examination under the microscope of swabs taken from the urethra and, when necessary, from the throat and rectum, will confirm the diagnosis. Treatment with antibiotics is usually effective and should be given to all sexual partners. Left untreated, gonorrhoea may spread to infect the testicles or prostate gland. Arthritis and blood poisoning are other possible complications.

Trichomoniasis

This STD is caused by a single-cell parasite which may invade and multiply inside the urethra and under the foreskin (in uncircumcised men), occasionally spreading to the prostate gland. Symptoms of trichomoniasis in men may include discomfort on passing urine and a yellowish-green urethral discharge. Many men who are exposed to this infection do not have symptoms and there is no discharge to examine for parasites under the microscope. Nevertheless, if your female sexual partner has been diagnosed as suffering from trichomoniasis you should be treated with the antibiotic metronidazole to avoid the risk of re-infecting her in the future.

Thrush

This common yeast infection may be passed on through sexual intercourse with an infected partner, but in most cases it starts for reasons other than sexual activity. Symptoms, including redness and itchiness at the end of the penis, are treated with an antifungal cream. Thrush is more common in women, and a man is unlikely to be the cause of his female partner's thrush. However, if your partner does develop symptoms, it is still worth using an antifungal cream for at least a week, just in case.

Syphilis

Infection with spirochaetes, the spiral-shaped bacteria that cause syphilis, results in the appearance of a painless sore or ulcer (chancre) on the penis, mouth or anus two or three weeks later. The diagnosis is confirmed by examining cells scraped from the surface of this chancre under a microscope. Left untreated, the chancre usually heals up, but the infected individual then enters the second stage of syphilis (which may be a few weeks or a few months later or may even overlap with the first stage), with the development of a fever, headache, rash and enlarged lymph nodes. A blood test will confirm the infection.

Antibiotic treatment, usually an injection of penicillin, eradicates syphilis in most cases. However, regular blood tests are needed over the following two years to make absolutely sure the infection does not recur. If syphilis is not treated in the first or second stage, there is a good chance that the infection will come back many years after the symptoms have disappeared, causing damage to many body organs and tissues, including the heart, aorta, brain and nervous system.

Genital herpes

This STD is caused by a virus, similar to the herpes virus that results in cold sores. An attack of genital herpes characteristically begins with itching or tingling around or on the genitals, followed by the eruption of painful, fluid-filled blisters. These blisters start off clear, turn yellow and then burst, before drying to form scabs that heal slowly.

An initial attack of genital herpes may last up to three weeks; the virus then remains dormant in the genital tissues, causing recurrent symptoms in more than half the men who have been exposed to it. In addition to the painful blistering, there may also be headaches, 'flu symptoms and swollen lymph nodes.

On average, genital herpes will flare up about five times a year, although attacks tend to become less frequent and less severe with age. Treatment with the antiviral drug acyclovir can speed up healing of the blisters and reduce the number of attacks. A warm salt-water bath can ease the discomfort associated with the blistering, but strong painrelievers may also be required.

To avoid picking up or passing on genital herpes, there should be no sexual contact during an attack. A condom will reduce the risk of spreading this infection during sexual intercourse, but it is not a fail-safe measure.

Genital warts

Genital warts may appear anywhere on the penis or around the anus; they can also grow out of sight inside the urethra or anal canal, in which case the only symptom may be an itch or painless irritation. When they are visible, these warts appear as small bumps or lumps, usually coloured pink or red and growing singly or in clusters. Some are smooth, some are shaped like the outside of a cauliflower.

After someone has been exposed to the human papilloma virus that causes genital warts, the growths may appear at any time over the next few months. They are usually treated by applying the chemical solution podophyllin (available on prescription) to kill the virus and washing it off a few hours later. Never use any of the ordinary wart-removers from the pharmacist as they are likely to cause pain and irritation. Occasionally, several applications of podophyllin are needed and, if the warts persist, surgical removal may be required.

Once a doctor has checked that the warts have cleared, sexual activity may be resumed. However, genital warts often grow back and need further treatment. Any female partner of a man who has been diagnosed as suffering from genital warts will be advised to have an annual cervical smear because of the proven link between exposure to the wart virus and cervical cancer. A male partner should go to an STD clinic for a check-up as well, even if he does not have any obvious genital warts.

Pubic lice (crabs)

These small, brown, wingless, crab-like creatures, about 2mm long, are usually spread from one person to another during sexual contact, although simply being naked and close to someone with this infection puts you at risk.

Pubic lice latch on to hairs in the genital region and feed off blood by biting the skin. In hairy men, the lice may also be found around the anus. Minute white eggs may be produced by the females and the biting may cause irritation.

Treatment involves application of an insecticide solution (available from the pharmacist) to the infected hairy areas, which is usually left on for up to 24 hours before being washed off. Sexual partners must also be treated and all bed linen should be washed at a temperature of at least 60°C.

Hepatitis B

This potentially fatal liver disease is caused by infection with a virus which can be carried in all body fluids, including semen, saliva, vaginal fluids and blood. Although hepatitis B does not affect the sexual organs, sexual intercourse is one way in which the virus is passed from one person to another. It is also able to survive outside the body for several days in dried blood and on a variety of exposed surfaces. It can be spread by injecting drug users sharing a contaminated needle, as

HIV can be, but, unlike HIV, it can also be caught from, for example, an infected toothbrush or razor.

About half of the people who become infected with hepatitis B develop acute inflammation of the liver several weeks or even months later. Symptoms may include loss of appetite, nausea, vomiting, weakness, fatigue, joint pains and jaundice. Many sufferers mistake this illness for an attack of 'flu; others are too ill to do anything but rest in bed, and take months to recover.

Unlike many other STDs, hepatitis B has no cure. Medication may be prescribed to relieve symptoms and to control the effects of any liver damage, but the disease itself has to be allowed to run its own course. In the meantime, the usual advice is to rest in bed, not to drink any alcohol and not take any other drug that has to be processed by the liver.

About ten per cent of hepatitis B sufferers go on to develop a chronic form of the disease, regardless of the severity of the original infection; even though they don't have any symptoms, these 'silent carriers' can still pass on the disease to others. In addition, many carriers subsequently develop liver cancer, or liver failure due to cirrhosis.

It is not only people with chronic hepatitis B that can spread the infection without knowing about it: the virus can also be passed on even before the initial symptoms have appeared. However, the good news is that there is an effective vaccine to protect against hepatitis B and this is recommended for anyone whose job or lifestyle is likely to put them in contact with the virus, including medical and nursing staff, police and prison warders, homosexuals and heterosexuals with multiple partners, prostitutes, intravenous drug users and any family contacts of these people.

HIV and AIDS

HIV – Human Immunodeficiency Virus – infection may be passed on from one person to another in several different ways:

- by unprotected intercourse (anal or vaginal) with someone who has previously been infected by HIV. If one partner is infected, unprotected anal intercourse carries a particularly high risk of transmitting HIV, but unprotected vaginal intercourse also represents a significant risk

- through inoculation with, or transfusion of, infected blood or blood products. In the UK, since the introduction of improved screening of blood donors and the purifying treatment of plasma products, such as the clotting factor given to haemophiliacs, HIV is unlikely to be passed on in a transfusion. However, infected blood may be injected by a drug user who is sharing contaminated equipment. Also, there have been many cases of dentists, doctors, nurses and laboratory technicians being exposed to HIV when a needle or other instrument has accidentally punctured their skin, although very few have actually become HIV-positive (*see below*)
- a mother may pass HIV to her baby in the womb, during the delivery, or through breastfeeding.

Although most of the people who have HIV in Britain are homosexuals or injecting drug users (groups recognised as having high-risk behaviour), the fastest-growing group of sufferers have contracted HIV through heterosexual intercourse. It is, however, important to realise that the virus cannot be transmitted simply through casual social contact, for example, touching, cuddling or shaking hands. Nor is HIV passed on by coughing, sneezing, getting an insect bite or from being a blood donor. It is also perfectly safe to share cutlery, crockery, towels and toilet seats.

Symptoms of HIV

This virus invades white blood cells and multiplies inside them. Any time between three weeks and three months after exposure to HIV, symptoms similar to glandular fever (*see pages 199–200*) may develop, with a high temperature, headache and swollen lymph nodes. These symptoms usually disappear, enabling most people with HIV to continue leading normal lives with no obvious effects on their physical health.

Because HIV results in the formation of specific antibodies to the virus (in which case the person is referred to as HIV-positive), the diagnosis may be made from a blood test. It may take three months for these antibodies to appear and so a negative test result is only relevant if that individual has avoided all high-risk activity for at least three months before the test.

Once an adult is confirmed as being HIV-positive, the antibodies won't go away, but he or she may remain in good health for many years. Currently in the UK the average time for HIV infection to progress to AIDS is 8–10 years. People who are found to be HIV-positive should take extra care of their health by eating a varied balanced diet, following a regular exercise routine and using relaxation techniques to prevent a build-up of stress. All of these measures will help them stay healthy for longer. They should also take every reasonable precaution to avoid passing HIV on to others.

AIDS and associated illnesses

AIDS – Acquired Immune Deficiency Syndrome – may develop suddenly in someone who has for years been HIV-positive. Sometimes, this progression of the disease is preceded by symptoms such as diarrhoea, weight loss, night sweats and swollen lymph nodes, a phase known as AIDS-related complex.

The onset of AIDS may result in a variety of diseases, most of which are due to the virus causing failure of the body's immune defences against infection and cancer. People with AIDS become more susceptible to infections such as thrush, shingles, herpes, TB, Kaposi's sarcoma (a rare form of skin cancer) and pneumocystis carinii (an unusual type of pneumonia).

Antiviral drugs, such as zidovudine (AZT), may slow down the progress of AIDS in some people, but they can also cause serious side-effects. At present, doctors have to concentrate primarily on treating each complication as it develops because there is as yet no treatment for HIV. Death is usually due to one of these complications rather than to HIV.

AIDS and HIV information

The National AIDS Helpline* provides a free 24-hour service of advice and counselling on HIV and AIDS for all members of the public. The Terrence Higgins Trust* provides a range of services, including a helpline, for people with HIV and AIDS, their families and partners. This charitable organisation can also provide information on self-help groups and other resources which are available in different parts of the UK.

Contraception

There are many different methods of contraception to choose from. Although the male condom is the only contraceptive currently available for which the man can be directly responsible, it is still important for men to be aware of the advantages and disadvantages of other forms of contraception. That way he can be involved in deciding which method would be most suited to both his and his partner's needs, and the mutual support and shared responsibility can only benefit the relationship.

No contraceptive is absolutely fail-safe and all have some disadvantages. It is important to discuss the options in terms of their effectiveness, safety and convenience and to remember the principles of safer sex described earlier; even if the Pill or coil is the woman's first choice of contraceptive in the early stages of a relationship, it is still wise to use a barrier method, such as the male condom, to prevent the possible transmission of STDs such as HIV.

Advice on contraception may be obtained from a GP, family planning clinic or Brook Advisory Centre* (for young couples aged 25 years or under).

Male condom

The male condom consists of a sheath of thin latex rubber, usually lubricated to make it easier to roll on to the erect penis. Those few men who are allergic to the latex in a condom are usually able to tolerate a special low-allergy brand. Used properly, the male condom is extremely effective, with only two pregnancies per year for every 100 couples relying on this method alone. The number of pregnancies is much higher when the instructions are not followed correctly.

In addition to its contraceptive efficiency, male condoms protect against the transmission of herpes, genital warts, chlamydia and HIV. Men who tend to suffer from premature ejaculation may find that the condom helps by slightly reducing sensory stimulation. The male condom is not suitable for men who often temporarily lose their erection during intercourse, as the condom is likely to slip off.

Because sperm may be present in the lubricating secretions released prior to ejaculation, the condom should always be put on before any genital contact.

Squeezing the tip of the condom while it is being put on prevents air being trapped, which might otherwise increase the risk of it bursting. It is also important not to catch the condom on a fingernail, which might tear it. Before using a condom for the first time, it may be worth practising with one when masturbating to get used to putting it on and taking it off.

After orgasm, but before the erection has completely subsided, your penis should be withdrawn from your partner's vagina. The rim of the condom should be held against your penis to prevent it slipping off and accidentally spilling semen. If penetration lasts longer than ten minutes, it is also a good idea to withdraw to check the condom hasn't been damaged. Never re-use a condom.

A condom may be weakened within seconds of coming into contact with any oil-based lubricant, such as baby oil or Vaseline, so only water-based lubricants, such as KY jelly, should be used. If a massage oil has been used prior to sex, the hands should be wiped before the condom is touched.

Condoms are now on sale in supermarkets, petrol stations and by mail order, as well as in more traditional locations such as pharmacies, barbers' and slot machines found in public toilets. Various types of condom – including coloured, ribbed, shaped and flavoured – are available, but only those with a safety kitemark have a guarantee of quality.

Female condom

This relatively new type of barrier contraceptive consists of a large tube made of very thin polyurethane plastic or rubber with two flexible rings, one at each end, to hold it in place. The ring at the closed end fits inside the vagina while the ring at the open end stays outside, lying flat against the entrance to the vulva and vagina.

During intercourse, you should make sure that your penis passes into the condom and not around it; your partner may need to guide you in during initial penetration. The condom may move during sex, but sperm won't escape into the vagina as long as the penis remains inside the condom. After orgasm the outer ring of the female condom should be twisted to ensure that the ejaculated semen is retained, then the condom should be gently pulled out.

In addition to protecting against pregnancy, the female condom should also prevent the spread of STDs, but this is still to be proved scientifically.

Some women are initially put off by the large size of the female condom – it measures over 17 × 7cm – but these are the actual dimensions of the inside of the vagina. If your partner finds it difficult to fit the female condom at first, she will find it becomes easier with practice. Because it can be put in before intercourse, one advantage is that it does not interrupt love-making. Also, many men find it allows for greater stimulation than the male condom.

Spermicides

Substances which chemically destroy sperm are available as creams, jellies, foams and pessaries. Used on their own, these spermicides are not very effective and if foam or a pessary needs to be inserted into the woman's vagina, this has to be done at least 30 minutes before intercourse to allow it time to dissolve and become active. Some condoms are impregnated with a spermicide to offer additional protection and a spermicide can also be used in combination with a diaphragm or cap for the same reason. There is also evidence to suggest that a spermicide may kill HIV.

Contraceptive sponge

An alternative barrier method of contraception, which uses a spermicide, is the vaginal sponge. This disposable circular polyurethane foam sponge, impregnated with the spermicide nonoxyl-9, is first moistened with water and then pushed high into the woman's vagina before intercourse. One side of the sponge has an indentation that fits over the cervix to form a barrier.

The sponge must be left in place for at least six hours after sex, although it remains effective for up to 24 hours. A loop is attached to the sponge to make it easier to remove, after which it should be thrown away. Even used correctly, the contraceptive sponge is not as effective as either the male or the female condom.

Diaphragm and cap

A diaphragm is a hemispherical dome of thin rubber, with a coiled metal spring inside the rim, which fits diagonally behind the cervix across the front wall of the vagina and extends to the bony ledge at the front of the pelvis. The cervical cap is a smaller, more rigid rubber device which fits snugly over the opening into the uterus by suction.

The family planning doctor will first find the size of diaphragm or cap that fits the woman comfortably. She will then be taught how to insert and remove it herself. A spermicide should be used with the diaphragm or cap to provide additional protection, with extra spermicide inserted into the vagina if intercourse occurs more than once while it is in.

Unlike the sponge, the diaphragm or cap can be used repeatedly. After sex, it should be left in the vagina for at least six hours to prevent any surviving sperm from reaching the uterus.

Oral contraceptive pill

The most commonly prescribed pill contains a combination of synthetic oestrogen and progesterone, which suppress the release of two pituitary gland hormones. As a result, the maturation of eggs inside the ovaries is inhibited and the release of an egg during each menstrual cycle (ovulation) is prevented. In addition to stopping ovulation, the combined pill also thickens the mucus produced by the cervix, making it more hostile to sperm; and it interferes with the development of the uterus lining, which normally happens during the second half of the cycle, to stop implantation just in case an egg is released and fertilised.

Another type of pill, the so-called mini pill, contains only synthetic progesterone. Although it doesn't always prevent ovulation, its effect on the cervical mucus and uterus lining is normally sufficient to prevent conception. The mini pill is less likely to cause side-effects than the combined pill, but its effectiveness depends on the woman taking it at almost the same time every day, whereas the timing of the combined pill can be less precise.

Your partner may be advised to take the mini pill rather than the combined pill if she is a heavy smoker, is breastfeeding or has a history of high blood pressure, high blood cholesterol, heart disease, migraine, thrombosis or liver disease.

Emergency contraception

If unprotected intercourse with your partner occurs, for example, as a result of a condom splitting or if she has forgotten to put in her diaphragm, it is possible to use an emergency method of contraception sometimes misleadingly referred to as the 'morning after' pill. Your GP or family planning clinic will provide your partner with four tablets, each containing oestrogen and progesterone, two tablets to take immediately and two as a second dose to be taken 12 hours later.

As long as these pills are started within 72 hours of unprotected intercourse, pregnancy can be prevented. Depending on the stage of your partner's menstrual cycle, this relatively high-dose pill will work either by preventing ovulation or by stopping the fertilised egg from implanting.

As another form of emergency contraception, an IUCD (*see below*) can be inserted up to five days after intercourse.

Vaginal ring

This silicone-based rubber ring has a hollow inner core filled with synthetic progesterone. Once inserted high in the vagina, the ring releases small amounts of progesterone continuously, thus having the same contraceptive action as the progesterone-only mini pill (*see above*).

The advantage of the vaginal ring is that there is no worry over having to take a pill at the same time every day; it is therefore a more reliable contraceptive than the mini pill. Your partner simply has to replace the ring every three months before the supply of progesterone begins to run out.

Intrauterine contraceptive device (IUCD)

An IUCD (coil) is a small plastic device, usually wrapped in thin copper wire, which is inserted inside the uterus by the GP or family planning clinic doctor. The contraceptive effect of an IUCD appears to come from the inflammation it causes inside the uterus, which creates a hostile environment for sperm, as well as making the lining of the uterus unreceptive to implantation of a fertilised egg.

Copper-containing IUCDs can usually be left in the uterus for between three and five years before they have to be replaced. A newer variety of IUCD, which also releases tiny amounts of synthetic progesterone to increase its contraceptive efficiency, has to be changed every 12 months.

Because of the increased risk of pelvic infection, which can lead to infertility, this method of contraception is normally recommended only for older women not planning to have any more children.

Hormone injections

Injections of a long-acting synthetic progesterone can have a reliable contraceptive effect for up to six months. However, this controversial method has generally been reserved for women who cannot cope with other types of contraceptive and has proved unpopular because of the high incidence of side-effects, such as irregular heavy periods and weight gain. Progesterone injections have recently been superseded by progesterone implants, which first became available in the UK at the end of 1993.

Hormone implants

Six thin, flexible capsules containing synthetic progesterone are inserted, under local anaesthetic, beneath the skin on the inside of the woman's upper arm. Tiny amounts of this hormone are released continuously into the bloodstream, resulting in the same contraceptive mechanism of action as the progesterone-containing mini pill and vaginal ring.

Clinical trials have shown that hormone implants are at least as effective a contraceptive as the combined pill and more effective than the mini pill and the various barrier methods of contraception. Whereas the progesterone ring has to be changed every three months, the implants remain active for a minimum period of five years. Irregular menstruation is the most common side-effect, but this usually resolves itself within six months.

Natural methods

Natural family planning works on the principle that sexual intercourse takes place only on the days of your partner's menstrual cycle which precede or follow her fertile phase (the rhythm method). However, to determine which days are unsafe it is necessary to predict when ovulation is occurring, which is easier said than done.

After ovulation, the human egg survives for a maximum of only 24 hours. Sperm are known to be capable of surviving for a maximum of seven days inside one of the fallopian tubes. Therefore, for conception to occur, sexual intercourse must take place within seven days of ovulation, or at some time during the 24 hours after ovulation – the fertile phase of the menstrual cycle.

Your partner can use several techniques to monitor the time at which she ovulates:

- one way is to record her body temperature first thing every morning, before eating, drinking, smoking or taking any exercise, and then to plot these daily readings on a chart. A sudden rise of about 0.5°C occurs at ovulation, a small change but enough to be a reliable predictor as long as the recordings are done correctly using a special fertility thermometer with an easy-to-read scale, and your partner has not for any reason developed a fever. The infertile or safe phase begins on the morning of the third consecutive higher temperature reading
- another sign of ovulation is a change in the cervical mucus, which becomes thicker and less elastic during the second half of the menstrual cycle (i.e. after ovulation)
- the cervix also characteristically feels firmer and moves down a little after ovulation.

Unfortunately, prediction of the exact time of ovulation before it occurs is virtually impossible. Although ovulation precedes the first day of menstruation by about 14 days, most women who aren't taking the contraceptive pill have variable menstrual cycles, so the actual timing of ovulation may differ from one month to the next by several days. As a result, the safe phase during the first half of the cycle can be highly unpredictable and carries a greater risk of pregnancy than the infertile phase after ovulation.

Natural family planning requires considerable self-discipline if you are to avoid sexual intercourse on your partner's fertile days. One solution is to use a condom at these times. If you use withdrawal as a contraceptive technique you are highly likely to end up with your partner pregnant, partly because sperm are known to be released in small numbers within the lubricating fluid that appears before ejaculation and also because you may fail to pull your penis clear of the vagina in time.

Sterilisation

Vasectomy

For couples who have decided that they do not want to have any more children, sterilisation of the man by vasectomy is a simple, relatively safe and highly effective procedure. This operation is usually carried out under a local anaesthetic, after which the man can go straight home. Evidence of the popularity of vasectomy comes from the fact that this method of fertility control is now relied on by over half a million couples in the UK.

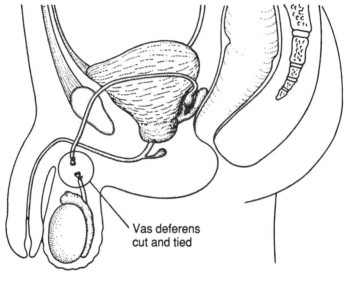

Vas deferens
cut and tied

Vasectomy

Considering vasectomy

If you are considering having a vasectomy, you must be as sure as you can be that you have completed your family and will not want any more children under any circumstances. Vasectomy should be regarded as a permanent method of contraception that cannot be reversed.

Before the surgeon agrees to perform a vasectomy, he or she will ensure that someone – usually your GP or a specialist counsellor – has explained the significance of the procedure to you and given you the opportunity to discuss the implications. Ideally, your partner should also be involved in this counselling process, although it is not essential.

It is possible for young men to have a vasectomy, but they are likely to be encouraged to spend longer thinking through their options before confirming their decision. Certainly, any man who admits to going through personal or sexual difficulties at the time he is requesting a vasectomy will be advised against having the operation.

Waiting lists for a vasectomy on the NHS may be several months long in some parts of the UK. However long the wait, it is important for couples to continue using some form of reliable contraception in the meantime. A vasectomy done privately will cost about £150–£250.

The vasectomy operation

Before the operation, any hair on your scrotum will usually be shaved off so that it doesn't get caught up in the stitches. You will probably be asked to shave yourself. After the scrotal skin has been cleaned with antiseptic, a local anaesthetic will be injected under the skin and around each vas deferens (the two tubes that connect each testicle to the urethra). This may cause a slight stinging sensation before the tissues become numb.

Once the anaesthetic has taken effect, one or two small cuts will be made in the skin of the scrotum to reveal the vas deferens. A small piece of each vas deferens is then cut out and the ends either side of the cut bent back and tied with stitches. Throughout this procedure you should not feel any pain, only a pulling sensation (usually in the lower abdomen). To ensure each vas deferens has been correctly identified and cut, the two sections that have been removed may be sent off to the laboratory for examination under a microscope.

Dissolvable stitches are generally used to close the scrotal incision, which is then covered with a sterile dressing. To reduce the amount of discomfort and swelling, you will usually be provided with a scrotal support or advised to wear close-fitting underpants or swimming trunks for a few days. Some men feel faint after a vasectomy, but this sensation usually goes away within 15 minutes.

Recovering from a vasectomy

On the day of the vasectomy, you should go home and take things easy. However, the following day most men are fit enough to return to work as long as their job does not involve strenuous exercise, heavy lifting or driving for long distances. These specific types of activity, and sports that require running or jumping, are best avoided for a week, or at least until the wound discomfort has passed.

Ordinary painrelievers, such as aspirin or paracetamol, should be enough to control any discomfort after a vasectomy, which will usually ease off anyway within a few days. You should wash your scrotum gently in the shower or bath from the day after the operation.

Complications after a vasectomy are extremely rare. There may be some bruising and swelling, but these should disappear within a week or two. Occasionally the wound becomes infected and has to be treated with antibiotics; or a small blood clot forms to cause a painful swelling that has to be removed surgically. The wound itself should have healed completely within ten days and any scar left behind is usually invisible.

Sex after a vasectomy

Sexual intercourse can begin again as soon as the discomfort in your scrotum eases off, but there may be a slight pain associated with ejaculation on the first few occasions. Until all the sperm stored inside the vas deferens have been used up, you are still potentially fertile and must continue with your usual method of contraception until two consecutive semen samples checked in the laboratory have been found to be free of sperm.

The time it takes for all the sperm in each vas deferens to disappear varies between different men, but it usually requires at least ten ejaculations to clear them completely. You will normally be asked to provide a semen sample by masturbation 12 and 14 weeks after the vasectomy and sometimes after a minimum of 20 ejaculations. Further samples will be requested until they become free of any sperm.

Vasectomy should have no effect on orgasm, ejaculation or sexual performance. Semen will continue to be ejaculated. The sperm it would normally contain are still being produced in the testicles but are unable to pass along the vas deferens. They will simply be reabsorbed by the body.

A few men suffer temporary impotence after a vasectomy, which is due to psychological rather than physical factors. This problem usually disappears with reassurance and help from the man's partner to regain his sexual confidence. Occasionally, specialist counselling is needed and if this fails the procedure may have to be reversed.

Long-term complications

The chance of the cut ends of the vas deferens spontaneously rejoining is extremely rare. There have been one or two cases in the past of men getting their partners pregnant several years after a vasectomy, but with modern surgical techniques this is unlikely to happen.

Around half of the men who have had a vasectomy start to produce antibodies against their own sperm. However, this will only be a problem if they request a reversal of the procedure (whereby the cut ends of the vas deferens are rejoined) at a later date, with the aim of having another child.

Female sterilisation

Every year in the UK about 90,000 women are sterilised, having decided they do not want to have any more children. Female sterilisation, like a vasectomy, should be regarded as a permanent method of contraception that cannot be reversed and counselling will therefore be carried out before the operation, ideally with the woman's partner present as well. Some women are able to have their sterilisation reversed at a later date, but there is no guarantee that this will be successful.

Unlike a vasectomy, female sterilisation requires a general anaesthetic and your partner will usually have to remain in hospital overnight. The operation consists of blocking both fallopian tubes to stop eggs from reaching and thus being fertilised by sperm. No further contraception is needed following female sterilisation. Some women experience heavier periods after being sterilised, but it is not known how this is related to the operation as the uterus and ovaries are left intact.

Waiting lists for female sterilisation on the NHS may be as long as two years in some parts of the UK. In the meantime, some other form of contraception should be used. The cost of female sterilisation done privately is about £360.

Abortion

Making the decision to have an abortion and then going through with it can be an extremely traumatic experience for a woman. It is also a difficult time for the male partner, who may be experiencing a complex mixture of emotions but is much less likely to be given the opportunity to express his true feelings openly.

Counselling before an abortion can help reduce the emotional impact of terminating the pregnancy and is essential, regardless of whether the reason for the abortion is social, psychological, physical or because of an abnormality in the baby. Even a woman who has definitely made up her mind will find it useful to discuss her feelings with someone who is not emotionally involved with her or her pregnancy.

If your partner is about to have an abortion, it is important for you to show your support by offering to go with her to the doctor or counsellor. You will also benefit from being involved in the discussions. After the abortion, you should be prepared for your partner to go through a variety of emotions, which may include euphoria, anger, guilt, depression and a feeling of numbness, although she may just be relieved that the pregnancy is over. These reactions are perfectly normal, but if symptoms such as depression persist, or become more severe, further counselling and possibly medication may be required.

Making the arrangements

If your partner has decided she doesn't want to continue with her pregnancy, she should see her doctor as soon as possible. The earlier the abortion is performed, the less traumatic it is likely to be both physically and psychologically. Within nine weeks of conception it may be possible for her to be referred for the new abortion pill, avoiding the need for surgery. After 12 weeks it may be more difficult to get an abortion on the NHS in some parts of the UK. Abortions are carried out in NHS hospitals (free of charge) and in charitable or private clinics (where there will be a charge). If your partner doesn't want to be referred by her GP, she can be seen by the local family planning clinic doctor, or she can contact the charitable or private clinic directly.

For a woman to have an abortion, two different doctors must agree that she has reasonable grounds and sign an official form declaring which situation applies in her case. Sometimes the abortion is done because tests have shown the baby has severe abnormalities. However, the usual reason given is that continuing with the pregnancy may threaten the mother's physical or mental health, taking into account social circumstances such as personal relationships, existing children and housing.

Methods of abortion

Whichever technique is used, abortion done under proper medical supervision is a relatively safe procedure, with a low risk of complications, such as infection. Future problems with infertility or miscarriage are no more likely to occur in women who have had a previous abortion.

Abortion pill

Although this new form of medical abortion is licensed to be used in all hospitals and clinics where abortions are carried out, it is not routinely available on the NHS and, in any case, many women are referred for abortion after the nine-week limit.

Initially the woman is given pills which contain mifepristone (RU486), a drug which causes the uterus lining to break down by blocking the action of her progesterone hormones. Vaginal bleeding will usually begin at any time over the next 48 hours. The woman then returns to the hospital or clinic two days later and, if the pills haven't already terminated the pregnancy, she will have a pessary containing prostaglandin inserted into her vagina. This pessary will stimulate uterine contractions, which may be painful and accompanied by heavy bleeding, and the termination will be completed within six hours. The woman will then be allowed home, to return for a check-up seven days later.

Vacuum aspiration

The cervix is dilated and a tube is inserted into the uterus and connected to a suction pump to draw out the foetus and placenta. Occasionally, the uterus lining also has to be scraped clear using a sharp spoon-shaped instrument known as a curette.

Prostaglandin infusion

This technique, which may be necessary once a pregnancy passes beyond the 14th week, stimulates the uterus to contract and expel the foetus, rather like inducing labour. Contractions are powerful enough to require painrelievers. The procedure may take up to 24 hours and vaginal bleeding may continue for over a week afterwards.

Trying for a baby

If you and your partner have decided to start a family, you can increase your chance of success by making sure you have intercourse just before the time when your partner is due to ovulate. In contrast to the rhythm method of contraception, described on page 128, in which intercourse is restricted to the infertile phase of the woman's menstrual cycle, the focus of sexual activity is now the fertile phase.

At first, there is no need to worry about predicting the exact time of ovulation. Many couples successfully conceive within a few months by aiming to have sex every other day, particularly during the middle two weeks of the woman's menstrual cycle. However, if this proves unsuccessful, the next stage is to use one of the following techniques to find out when ovulation is occurring.

- If your partner's menstrual cycle is regular, count back 14 days from the day menstruation would be expected to start.
- Your partner should check her temperature each morning using the method described on page 129 to find out when ovulation has taken place. Keeping a temperature chart over several months will generally reveal a consistent pattern and allow ovulation to be predicted before rather than after it actually occurs.
- Your partner may notice that her cervical mucus increases in volume and becomes thinner, clearer and more elastic just before she ovulates, allowing her to stretch an unbroken thread of it between her thumb and forefinger.
- An ovulation-predictor kit can be bought from the pharmacist without a prescription, but these kits tend to be expensive. Your partner can then test her urine, looking for a particular colour change which indicates the presence of a hormone released 24–36 hours prior to ovulation.

Help with conception

A recent survey revealed that only half the couples who had been trying for a baby were successful within the first six months. Another quarter of the couples took a year to conceive and one in five of the remainder had to wait up to two years. You should not, therefore, expect your partner to become pregnant as soon as you stop using contraception. Some delay is normal and does not mean that one or both of you has a problem.

If you have been having unprotected sex regularly (two to three times a week) for over a year without success then you should make an appointment to see a doctor. It is essential that both partners are investigated at the same time because a fertility problem is just as likely to lie with the man as with his partner. Of the estimated one in six couples who are either infertile or having difficulty achieving pregnancy, statistics show that the cause lies with the male in 30 per cent of cases, the female in a further 30 per cent and in the remaining 40 per cent of cases there is either a combination of factors or no cause is ever found.

Some men wrongly assume that if they can get an erection and ejaculate, they are automatically fertile. This is not true, so you should not expect your partner to go through fertility tests on her own. Also, just because you have already fathered children during a previous relationship, for example, doesn't mean you are still fertile.

The doctor is likely to ask all sorts of questions about you and your partner's health and sexual activity, as well as carrying out an examination of your testicles. He or she will want to check that you have been having sex during your partner's fertile phase and will be on the lookout for possible reasons for a fertility problem, such as a history of infection involving the testicles or the presence of a varicocele (varicose vein in the scrotum).

Some of the basic investigations can be done by your GP: for example, sending a sample of your semen to the laboratory for analysis and getting your partner to keep basal body temperature charts for up to six months to check that she is ovulating and having sex just before ovulation.

Referral to a specialist

Before considering the various tests and treatments for infertility, it is important to be aware of the potential difficulties associated with obtaining the best or most appropriate specialist care. First, although there are NHS hospitals and clinics which offer infertility investigations and treatments, waiting lists tend to be very long and some tests and procedures may not be available. Also, even on the NHS, some charges may be made because of the very high cost of certain treatments.

Some private fertility clinics are subsidised by specialist charities, but it is advisable to check two things before agreeing to receive treatment: the estimated cost and the chance of success. Ask about all the different charges, including the price of repeated cycles of treatment. For example, in vitro fertilisation may cost between £800 and £2,200 per cycle, with an additional £450 for the drugs used.

When comparing the success rates of different clinics, it is best to concentrate on the results for couples of similar age groups with similar problems and to ask for the 'take-home baby rates' per cycle of treatment, not just the pregnancy rates. Larger fertility centres tend to have better success rates, but even the best figures are below 20 per cent for some forms of assisted conception.

Information and support
You and your partner should be aware that undergoing tests and treatment for infertility can put a considerable strain on your relationship. It is essential that you support each other through what can be a highly emotional and stressful experience. You should talk honestly about your feelings, be prepared to become angry, frustrated, depressed or anxious at times, but be careful not to start blaming each other for your difficulties.

Fertility clinics generally provide a specially trained counsellor to help couples come to terms with these powerful emotions and to accept the prospect of not being able to have a child of their own. The treatment itself can be extremely demanding, particularly for the woman, and both partners will have to learn to be patient as many months may pass before they are able to move on to the next stage of the process, or to see whether a particular procedure has been successful.

For further information and to be put in contact with a local support group, there are two organisations, ISSUE★ (National Fertility Association) and CHILD★, run by people who understand the feelings and experiences of couples having difficulty conceiving. In addition, the Human Fertilisation and Embryology Authority★ can provide a list of IVF and artificial insemination centres in the UK.

Causes of male infertility

Scientists have discovered a significant deterioration in the quality of sperm over the last 50 years, the number of sperm in each millilitre of semen having almost halved. There has also been a large increase in the numbers of abnormal sperm and in the proportion of men who have sperm which are less mobile (reduced motility). Environmental pollution is one factor which is being blamed for this decline in male fertility.

However, despite this rather alarming trend, the majority of men are still producing sperm in sufficient numbers and of good enough quality to have no problem with their fertility. Abnormal sperm with excessively large heads, double heads or double tails generally make up less than 20 per cent of the ejaculate, and even when this rises to 50 per cent there should still be enough healthy sperm to achieve conception when everything else is working normally.

The possible causes of male infertility include:

- defects in sperm production, which may be due to a genetic or hormone abnormality, undescended testicles, an environmental factor such as radiation exposure, previous infection like mumps, or an injury
- defects in sperm function, with reduced or absent motility, or inability to penetrate the egg
- obstruction to ejaculation due to an anatomical abnormality, blockage of the vas deferens following an infection like gonorrhoea, or previous vasectomy
- failure of ejaculation, due to impotence, or damage following prostatic or other pelvic surgery
- immune system problems, whereby the man or his partner has started to produce antibodies which inactivate or kill his sperm.

Tests for male infertility

In addition to undergoing an examination of the testicles, you will be asked to produce a sample of semen for analysis in the laboratory. You should refrain from ejaculating for about three days before collecting your specimen to provide a sample that represents your best-quality sperm and semen. You will be given a container and, having obtained the sample by masturbating, should deliver it to the laboratory within a few hours, having kept it warm in the meantime.

The sample will be examined under a microscope to check the number of sperm, their shape and how well they move. If any abnormality is found, you will need to provide a second sample, about two weeks later, for a repeat analysis. This is because there can be a considerable natural variation in an individual's sperm count and quality. If, despite following the standard recommendations for improving the production and health of your sperm (*see pages 159–61*), the abnormality is persistent, you will be referred to a specialist in male infertility (in the UK, usually a urologist).

Additional, more sophisticated sperm tests have been developed over the last few years. These include assessing the ability of sperm to penetrate cervical mucus or to fuse with an egg, and seeing whether chemicals which kill sperm, known as free radicals, are being released in the semen. Other tests to establish the cause of male infertility may include checking the level of a specific hormone in the blood or urine, taking a special X-ray or scan of the testicles to detect a blockage in the vas deferens and, occasionally, examining a biopsy from one of the testicles under a microscope.

One way to see whether your sperm is able to move freely and easily through your partner's cervical mucus is the post-coital test. To do this, you have sex a day or so before ovulation, when the mucus should be at its thinnest and most receptive. Your partner then attends the clinic between six and 18 hours later. A sample of mucus is taken from around her cervix to check the survival and fitness of the sperm as they swim through it.

Treatment of male infertility

A few men abstain from sexual intercourse for several weeks at a time in the mistaken belief that this will boost their sperm numbers and quality. In fact, it appears that regular intercourse at three- to four-day intervals gives the best chance of stimulating sperm production.

Treatment of infertility will depend on the specific cause, assuming one can be found. Hormone replacement therapy can help those few men found to have a hormonal abnormality. Surgical re-opening of a vas deferens blocked by scarring due to infection may restore fertility.

Reversal of a vasectomy is often technically successful, but sperm quality may be poor, usually because the vasectomy itself has resulted in the formation of antibodies against the man's own sperm. In men who have started to produce antisperm antibodies, steroid treatment may block this activity and thus enhance their fertility. A new technique, in which sperm are collected directly from the epididymis – this is known as microsurgical epididymal sperm aspiration (MESA) – is being used to try to overcome this antibody problem. However, MESA has proved largely unsuccessful because sperm are not fully mature until after they leave the epididymis.

Other new procedures to help overcome male infertility, done in conjunction with IVF, have been designed to counteract the problem of abnormal sperm motility which is thought to be preventing successful penetration of the egg. These techniques include the injection of a single sperm under the membrane around the egg (subzonal insemination or SUZI), or directly into the body of the egg

(ISCI or DISCO, depending on which of the two full names for this procedure is being abbreviated).

Preliminary results with these procedures appear promising, but they are still experimental and being tested in only a few British fertility centres. Sluggish sperm are also being treated with stimulants, similar to caffeine, to boost their motility.

Artificial insemination

In this process sperm are injected directly into a woman's cervix. Artificial insemination of a man's own sperm into his partner's cervix may be recommended if the male partner has a persistently reduced sperm count, for example, or where the sperm have difficulty penetrating his partner's cervical mucus. It may also be suggested if a physical disability prevents normal sexual intercourse.

Fresh sperm produced by masturbation are injected within as short a time as possible and the woman remains lying down with the foot of the bed raised for an hour or so afterwards. Insemination is timed to take place just before ovulation and is then repeated every two to three days to increase her chance of conception.

Insemination of sperm (kept frozen in a sperm bank) from a donor may be recommended if the man has no sperm, or a sperm count too low for artificial insemination or assisted conception, such as IVF, or if he is known to be a carrier for a particular genetic disease.

Counselling is recommended before donor insemination to make sure the man is completely comfortable about the idea of his partner carrying another man's baby. Although the donor remains anonymous, care is taken to match the male partner's physical characteristics, blood group and, if requested, his religion.

Female infertility

In addition to filling in a basal body temperature chart every day for several months to see whether there is an abrupt rise in mid-cycle that would suggest ovulation is occurring, your partner can undergo various other tests to find possible explanations for her difficulty in becoming pregnant:

- blood tests to identify a hormonal problem that may be interfering with ovulation

- an ultrasound scan to check her ovaries and uterus for disorders such as cysts and fibroids, and to confirm that an egg is being released from one of her ovaries at ovulation
- endometrial biopsy, in which a tiny sample of the woman's uterus lining is removed and examined under a microscope to make sure it is responding to hormonal changes, as well as being free of infection
- laparoscopy, a telescopic examination of her pelvic cavity to check for abnormalities in the shape and position of her uterus, to look for scarring of her fallopian tubes from infection or endometriosis and, by passing a blue dye up through her cervix at the same time, to see whether both fallopian tubes are free of obstruction
- X-rays, using a dye which shows up white, to confirm that her fallopian tubes are open.

Treatment of female infertility

If your partner is failing to ovulate each month, she may be prescribed a drug called clomiphene to take by mouth, as well as being injected with a synthetic hormone. Both of these measures stimulate the ovaries to ripen and release one or more eggs. Such drugs must be used extremely carefully to avoid too many eggs being released at the same time.

A blockage or scarring of the fallopian tubes may be corrected by surgical reconstruction, although this is usually successful only when the damage is slight. Women with more severe tubal damage can become pregnant only through an assisted conception technique, such as in vitro fertilisation (IVF).

IVF is not the answer to everyone's fertility problems, but, as well as helping overcome infertility due to blocked or absent fallopian tubes, it can also be successful if your sperm count is persistently low, or if your partner has developed sperm-killing antibodies. Also, there are some couples for whom IVF is successful even though the reason for their infertility has never been found.

To perform IVF, one or more mature eggs are removed from the woman's ovary and then combined outside her body with sperm from either her partner or a donor. The whole procedure is as follows:

- stimulation of ovulation using hormones
- monitoring maturation of the eggs in the ovary, using both ultrasound scanning and blood/urine measurements of the amount of oestrogen these eggs are producing

- injection of a hormone to complete the maturation of the eggs
- removal of the eggs from the ovary through a needle which is guided using ultrasound scanning
- fertilisation of eggs by sperm within a special growth material
- initial development of fertilised eggs in an incubator
- transferring no more than three embryos into the woman's uterus (once they are four to eight cells in size) through a thin tube guided into her cervix; any spares are kept frozen for a later treatment cycle
- pregnancy testing carried out 14 days later, along with an ultrasound scan to check that the tiny embryos have implanted in the uterus.

One large study of women who achieved a live birth after five IVF treatment cycles produced the following result: 45 per cent for those 34 years old and younger, 29 per cent if they were between 35 and 39, and only 14 per cent for those aged 40 to 45.

Women who need assisted conception but have normal fallopian tubes may be offered an alternative procedure known as gamete intrafallopian transfer (GIFT). The technique is basically the same as IVF, but it is cheaper and easier to perform; the sperm and eggs are kept separate and then transferred one after the other to one of the fallopian tubes, where fertilisation takes place. Any resulting embryo then travels naturally down into the uterus where implantation should occur. GIFT may be recommended if the woman's cervical mucus is hostile to her partner's sperm, or if there is no explanation for the couple's infertility.

Problems with intercourse

If you are suffering from a sexual problem, such as impotence or premature ejaculation, the first step is to overcome your embarrassment and discuss it with your partner, then, if necessary, seek professional help. The longer you delay visiting the doctor, counsellor or sex therapist, the more likely it is that your sexual difficulties will damage any long-standing relationship in which you are involved. Moreover, left untreated, sexual problems may cause depression or a build-up of anxiety, which will only make matters worse.

Your own GP may be one of the increasing number of doctors who have undertaken additional training in psychosexual therapy, and may therefore be able to offer help. Specialist sex therapy and counselling for sexual problems are also available on the NHS, but this service is very restricted in some parts of the UK and waiting lists are weeks, even months, long.

If you can afford to pay for private therapy, you could ask your GP to recommend a specialist, or you could contact either Relate★ (formerly the Marriage Guidance Council) or the British Association for Sexual and Marital Therapy★ for details of suitable sex therapists in your area. A number of good books are available, too, on the subject of sexual difficulties and how to overcome them.

The following section explains the possible causes of the most common psychosexual problems in men and gives some simple advice on self-help measures, as well as information on the sort of therapy that a specialist might recommend.

Reduced sex drive

Most men lose interest in sex at some time. This becomes a problem only if nearly every time your partner wants sex, you don't. Many different factors can reduce the sex drive (libido); the first step towards restoring an interest and appetite for sex is therefore to try to identify the most likely reasons.

Stress commonly reduces libido, particularly money worries, overwork, or fear of losing your job. Fatigue is another common reason, as is anxiety or depression. If you feel under stress, a regular relaxation exercise (*see* **Chapter 3**) and adjustment of your lifestyle will boost your emotional health, as well as your sex drive. When anxiety or depression is severe enough to interfere with your ability to live a normal life, including making love, it is time to ask your GP for help.

Not surprisingly, physical illnesses can also reduce libido, but, assuming the disease can be treated, an interest in sex should return as part of the recovery. Various drugs, such as blood pressure medication or sleeping tablets, can also lower the sex drive; your doctor should be able to suggest alternative medication.

Boredom may be a problem. The easy answer here, and the one that explains why so many marriages and partnerships break up every day, is to look for sexual excitement elsewhere. However, assuming you do want your relationship to work, there is much you can do to put the sparkle back in your sex life at home. For example, you should:

- talk to your partner about his or her sexual needs
- spend time stimulating your partner (and *vice versa*) before moving on to actual intercourse
- enjoy sex, not just the orgasm
- address any problems you and your partner are having outside the bedroom
- consider counselling if you and your partner are unable to talk over your difficulties yourselves.

Impotence

Impotence, being unable to get an erection or maintain an erection during sexual intercourse, is a fairly common sexual problem. Virtually all men will experience impotence at some time in their lives, usually only as a temporary reaction to something like stress, anxiety, fatigue, or drinking too much alcohol.

As men get older, they may notice that they require more intense or prolonged stimulation to achieve a satisfactory erection, as well as taking longer to become aroused again after ejaculation. Nevertheless, impotence should not necessarily be regarded as a normal part of ageing and men who are worried about this problem should seek medical help, regardless of their age.

If prolonged stress is the underlying cause of impotence, taking steps to reduce stress overload will usually help you relax enough to enjoy your sex life again. Treatment of depression, which may require some form of counselling in addition to antidepressant medication, can also restore sexual potency.

Various prescription drugs, including certain blood pressure treatments, antihistamines and sedatives, can cause impotence as one of their side-effects. In such cases you should check with your doctor to see whether switching to an alternative drug could help you. Smoking may increase the risk of impotence, as might alcohol abuse or any other type of recreational drug. Men who are overweight may boost their sexual performance by shedding a few kilograms, which may also improve their self-image and their self-confidence.

An abnormally low testosterone level could be the cause of impotence in some men, although this appears to be rare under the age of 65 (see male menopause, *pages 155–7*). Hormone replacement therapy, with testosterone, is usually prescribed only if tests have confirmed a deficiency of this sex hormone.

If you are suffering from impotence, it is also important to consider whether this is actually the result of problems in your relationship, rather than automatically blaming a physical disorder. You should try to discuss with your partner ways to vary your love-making, explaining what extra stimulation might help you achieve and maintain your erection. Oral sex is particularly effective at getting the blood flowing into the penis. Your doctor may suggest that you and your partner are referred to a sex therapist for counselling if you are having difficulty sorting out the problem.

Pelvic-floor muscle exercises, the routine women follow after childbirth to restore their vaginal tone and regain control of their urinary stream, can also help you improve your erection. You can practise this by stopping and starting the flow when passing urine.

One new method of dealing with impotence is the suction condom, worn during intercourse, which draws the penis erect in a similar way to the pressure applied during oral sex. A second type of vacuum sheath used prior to intercourse produces an erection which is then maintained by a silicone ring applied around the base of the penis.

Many urologists are now recommending self-injection of a drug that dilates blood vessels as a cure for impotence, including cases where the underlying cause is diabetes. Within 15 minutes of injecting this substance directly into the penis, using a simple device, an erection is produced and you will then be able to ejaculate as normal. Fortunately, this injection treatment is becoming easier to obtain on the NHS; the cost of a private consultation combined with the drug charges can add up to several hundred pounds. There is also a small risk of developing a painful prolonged erection, or tender scarring at the injection site.

When impotence cannot be reversed, for example, because of blood vessel and nerve damage, the only solution is surgical insertion of an artificial penile implant. As for injection therapy, referral for this procedure on the NHS may prove difficult. Also, although these implants are an effective way of achieving an erection, they occasionally become infected and have to be removed.

The simplest form of penile implant consists of two semi-rigid rods. Following surgery, the penis can be bent upwards for sexual intercourse and pointed downwards to conceal the erection at other times. However, the size of the penis will not alter during intercourse. There is also a hydraulic device which allows the penis to be inflated. Cylinders are implanted inside the penis and connected to a pump in the scrotum and a reservoir of fluid under the abdominal muscles. Squeezing the pump forces fluid from the reservoir into the cylinders to produce an erection; a release valve can be activated to return the fluid to the reservoir after intercourse, leaving the penis flaccid once again. The latest version is totally self-contained within the penis.

Pain during intercourse

Although dyspareunia (painful intercourse) is much more common in women than men, there are several medical disorders which can cause pain or discomfort for a man during sexual intercourse. If symptoms are interfering with your love life, you should make an appointment to see your doctor.

Possible causes of dyspareunia, all of which can be treated to relieve the discomfort, include balanitis (inflammation of the glans of the penis usually due to infection, but sometimes the result of an allergy to a spermicide or condom), phimosis (a tight foreskin) and Peyronie's disease (deformity of the penis due to scar tissue). These penis disorders are all discussed in more detail in **Chapter 6**. Inflammation of the prostate gland may sometimes cause stabbing pains at the tip of the penis, particularly during sexual intercourse.

Premature ejaculation

Occasional episodes of premature ejaculation, in which the man ejaculates almost immediately on, or even before penetration, occur in most men at some time in their love life. If you are anxious, the risk of your ejaculating prematurely increases, which is why it is more likely to happen when you are first having sex with a new partner. Unfortunately, even the worry that you might ejaculate before you have satisfied your partner is often enough to cause this common sexual problem.

The method usually recommended by sex therapists to help a man gain more control over ejaculation is the 'squeeze technique'. He asks his partner to firmly squeeze the head of his penis between his or her thumb and forefinger for a count of 10 each time he feels the urge to

147

ejaculate. This squeeze, which should not hurt, reduces the desire to ejaculate, allowing further stimulation to continue.

After practising the squeeze technique a few times during masturbation, you can try penetrative intercourse, withdrawing to have the penis squeezed each time you experience the sensations of impending ejaculation, until you feel ready to ejaculate. With patience and the co-operation of your partner, you should soon learn to hold back from ejaculating, without needing to stop for a squeeze.

Delayed ejaculation

Ejaculation in men occurs as a reflex response to continued stimulation of the erect penis. Occasionally, ejaculation does not happen, regardless of how long sexual intercourse continues, a condition known as delayed ejaculation. For most men, an isolated episode of delayed ejaculation has a simple explanation – they may have drunk too much alcohol, may be tired, may find a particular brand of condom is making intercourse less stimulating, or may already have ejaculated recently.

If you suffer from delayed ejaculation as a recurrent or continuous problem, you may have some underlying anxiety, of which you are not aware, about ejaculating into your partner . This may be related to a strict upbringing, hostile feelings towards your partner, or even the fear of a female partner becoming pregnant. To resolve these deep-rooted emotions, you and your partner may need counselling from a specially trained therapist.

The method usually recommended by sex therapists to help someone overcome the problem of delayed ejaculation is for a man to have intercourse until his partner is satisfied, then to withdraw his penis so that stimulation can be continued by masturbation. When the sensation of impending ejaculation is experienced, penetration is resumed so that ejaculation into his partner is inevitable. With the co-operation of their partners, most men find that after ejaculating during penetration on several occasions they start to find this much easier to do, without needing to stop for additional manual stimulation.

Homosexuality

Alfred C. Kinsey, an American sex expert, carried out a survey among over 4,000 white American adult men in the late 1940s which revealed that about four per cent were exclusively homosexual. A similar incidence of male homosexuality has been found in subsequent surveys conducted in the UK and continental Europe, as well as in the USA. However, at the time of writing a new survey by Kaye Wellings et al had just been published which suggested that of nearly 19,000 people interviewed in 1990–1 the incidence of exclusive homosexuality in men was much lower – closer to one per cent.

Homosexual encounters are common in adolescent boys coming to terms with their sexuality. They are generally regarded as a normal part of sexual development and are certainly nothing to feel guilty or upset about. In their teens, boys tend to develop intense relationships with other boys, regardless of whether they are in a mixed school or not. This bonding may include physical attraction and can lead to sexual contact, usually in the form of mutual masturbation.

The proportion of men who have experienced some form of homosexual activity at some stage in their life is thought to be about one in ten. Predictably, this figure is even higher in an environment such as a prison, where men are forced to live together without hetero-sexual contact. Homosexual relationships under these circumstances fulfil the need for an emotional outlet as well as relieving sexual tension. However, heterosexuals usually return to heterosexual activity as soon as the opportunity arises again.

Men who remain sexually attracted to both men and women all their lives, and whose erotic fantasies are almost equally divided between men and women, are in the minority. Men who appear to be bisexual because they are married or living with a female partner are in fact invariably homosexual – they may have married or moved in with a female partner before they discovered they were gay. Also, a number of men persevere with a heterosexual relationship in an attempt to deny their homosexuality, to disguise it from others or in response to pressure to conform socially.

A heterosexual relationship may continue because of the love and affection the homosexual man feels for his female partner, even if that love is not satisfying his physical and erotic desires. However, it may be best for the man to 'come out' to his female partner, regardless of the original motivation behind their relationship, out of respect for her as well as for the selfish reason of assisting the development of his own sexual identity. When and how he goes about revealing his homo-sexuality depends very much on his individual circumstances.

Finally, it is important to distinguish between the desire for physical contact with other men and contact which has sexual connotations. Many men hold back from touching or hugging another man because they worry that this will be misinterpreted as latent homosexuality.

Defining homosexuality

Male homosexuality is more than just a physical attraction to another man. Broadly speaking, it is a preference for emotional and physical contact with men rather than women, for example, when a man responds erotically to other men or has sexual fantasies about other men. It does not necessarily include any sexual activity with men.

Whatever fixed images and stereotypes the media may try to put across, homosexuals are as highly individual in their sexuality and relationships as are heterosexuals. Only a few display 'camp', overtly feminine behaviour and mannerisms.

Homosexual relationships do not necessarily involve anal intercourse (legal in the UK only between consenting males over the age of 18). There are many other ways in which two men can give each other sexual pleasure. While it is true that homosexual men are more likely than heterosexuals to have random, casual sexual encounters, this is not characteristic of all homosexual males. It is also important to remember that promiscuity is common among heterosexual males.

'Coming out'

For some young men, homosexual feelings and attractions are not just a phase they are going through as part of their sexual development. Realisation of their homosexuality will usually occur at some time between the ages of eight and 14. While many homosexual men are unable to remember their first same-sex erotic impulses or fantasies, they often recall certain behavioural characteristics which set them apart from their peers: for example, they may have avoided aggressive play or felt themselves to be more sensitive than other boys.

It can be extremely difficult for a young man to acknowledge his homosexuality. Even though it is being increasingly accepted as an alternative lifestyle, society's attitudes having become steadily more liberal over the past 20 years, there is still a great deal of hostility, intolerance, discrimination towards and oppression of homosexual men. A homosexual adolescent may try to deny his sexuality initially because of fears of persecution, teasing or bullying, for example. Later in life, he may be worried about it affecting his chances of getting a job.

Unfair treatment of homosexual men has been made worse by the AIDS epidemic (*see pages 113–4 and 120–2*), homosexuals having been falsely accused of being solely responsible for the existence and spread of the infection. Other common myths which encourage homophobic attitudes are that homosexual men are sexually aggressive or that they are more likely to molest children – accusations that are completely untrue.

With all this prejudice, it is not surprising that homosexual men sometimes try to suppress their true sexuality. Rather than making their lives easier, however, this denial leads to greater stress and unhappiness. Only when a homosexual man has learnt to love and respect himself as a homosexual can he go on to develop his sexual identity and form satisfactory relationships with other men. Continued denial is likely to lead to depression, isolation, alienation and a progressive erosion of self-esteem.

Often, an important step towards coming to terms with his homosexuality is for a man to 'come out' to his parents. They may initially be upset by the news, but this reaction may reflect their concern for his future happiness and well-being rather than being a sign that they don't unconditionally love their son. In some cases, rather than confronting his parents with his homosexuality, he may simply prefer not to disguise the fact to allow them to come to terms with it in their own way.

Although coming out is a highly individual experience, it can be facilitated by involvement in gay social networks. These make it easier to form non-sexual and sexual relationships with other gay men. For some men, confusion about their true sexuality can last for several years, but they can be reassured that there is no need to decide immediately where their preferences lie.

Explaining male homosexuality

Some doctors and psychologists try to explain away homosexuality as a pathological condition which, once the cause has been identified, can be treated and even 'cured'. For example, there have been some attempts to explain homosexuality in terms of emotional conditioning and a particular type of parenting during childhood.

Much has been written about the influence of specific parent models in determining the subsequent sexuality of a male child. It has been suggested that a powerful mother who has an intense relationship with her son can undermine his masculinity and inhibit the development of his sexual independence, and that a weak, detached or non-existent relationship with his father will make it even more difficult for the son to separate emotionally from his domineering mother. However, most homosexual men come from a normal home environment and, besides, unsatisfactory parental relationships also apply to large numbers of heterosexual men. In reality, such disruption of emotional development during childhood or adolescence is more likely to affect a man's ability to form sexual relationships of any kind than to influence his sexual orientation.

In the past, psychologists have even tried to use aversion therapy to convert a homosexual into a heterosexual man. It was thought that by giving an electric shock to a man each time he responded to an erotic picture of a male (but not when pictures of females were shown), he would learn to associate male erotica with pain and change his sexual preference as a result. Not surprisingly, aversion therapy failed to work in the long term and also risked seriously damaging the self-image of the man by reinforcing the perception that society regards homosexuality as undesirable.

Biological differences

The possibility of there being a biological difference between heterosexual and homosexual men has been the subject of a considerable amount of research. No evidence has been found, however, of any significant differences in the levels of the male sex hormone testosterone.

A study published in the American journal *Science* (30 August 1991) reported that a comparison of brain samples taken from heterosexual and homosexual men who died of AIDS showed a significant difference in the average size of a particular cell structure (INAH 3) inside the hypothalamus – the gland at the base of the brain which is associated with emotional response. The author of the study, Le Vay of the Salk Institute in Southern California, has argued that this difference is the result of hormonal action while the baby is developing inside his mother's womb. However, it may be that these changes are a consequence rather than a cause of an individual's sexual orientation. Also, other factors may influence this structure.

Finally, there has been a tremendous amount of publicity surrounding the possible existence of a 'gay gene'. Also in *Science* (16 July 1993), an American team of scientists reported the discovery of genetic markers on the tip of the X-chromosome – the sex chromosome inherited from the mother – which appear to be strongly linked to being homosexual. This study (carried out by Dr Dean Hamer and colleagues at the National Cancer Institute in Washington) was based on a detailed examination of the genetic make-up of over 100 homosexual men and their family trees. It is now hoped that the exact gene or genes which predispose a man to homosexuality can be identified.

The concept of a genetic basis to homosexuality continues to be heavily criticised in some quarters. If there does turn out to be a gay gene, this should only further emphasise that homosexuality in a man is as much a part of his persona as the colour of his hair or eyes, not a disorder that needs treatment.

Sexual deviation

Sexual deviation is any form of behaviour or activity that goes beyond what is regarded as socially acceptable and can be any of a variety of sexual practices which in no way enhance the love and affection that individuals feel for one another within a relationship. Most men who experience deviant sexual urges are uncertain of their masculinity; many, having failed to form any normal fulfilling sexual relationship with women or other men, feel sexually inadequate as a result. There also seems to be a tendency for adults who were sexually abused as children either to begin sexually deviant behaviour that involves abuse of others, or to continue being victims of abuse in adulthood.

Examples of sexual deviation include:

- voyeurism, whereby arousal is achieved by secretly watching other people have sex or get undressed, often accompanied by masturbation
- exhibitionism, in which exposure of the genitals to unsuspecting women causes sexual excitement, again often accompanied by masturbation, although only rarely associated with violence towards a victim

- transvestism, which means dressing in the clothes of the opposite sex to gain pleasure and often sexual excitement
- frottage, whereby a man becomes aroused by rubbing his genitals against a woman's body while pushed together in a crowd
- urophilia (or coprophilia), in which sexual excitement is a response to being urinated on (or defecated on)
- bestiality, which is sexual activity or intercourse with an animal
- sadism (or masochism), in which sexual arousal results from cruelty or violence towards (or from) someone
- fetishism, which becomes deviant behaviour when an individual experiences more sexual excitement with the fetish (object) than with its owner
- paedophilia, which is sexual activity or intercourse with a child.

Men who are prepared to seek treatment to control sexually deviant behaviour may respond well to psychosexual counselling, psychotherapy, or therapy from a psychologist which focuses on substituting alternative patterns of sexual behaviour that are socially acceptable. A GP should be able to recommend a suitable therapist without making any moral judgement about the sexual urges or fantasies described.

Sexual identity problems

One man in every 30,000 desperately wants to change his male sexual characteristics for those of a female, and to live his life as a woman. Transsexualism has nothing to do with homosexuality (sexual attraction to people of the same sex) or with transvestism (*see above*). A transsexual man feels he was born into the wrong body, and will want to dress as a woman, permanently and as a natural response to his desire to become a female.

Research into the cause of transsexualism suggests that sexual identity is determined primarily by the way a man was treated by his parents when he was a child. If a boy's parents subconsciously or consciously wanted a girl, then there is a greater chance that he will grow up unhappy with his sexual identity than if his parents had consistently treated him as a boy. This emotional conditioning is obviously a powerful phenomenon as it can override the genetic and hormonal factors that normally determine male sexual identity.

Before a transsexual man is considered for sex-change surgery, he will usually have to demonstrate that he has been successfully living as a woman for at least two years. A psychiatrist will check there is no significant mental disorder, such as schizophrenia. The man will then be referred to a gender reassignment programme, which includes counselling on dress and behaviour, as well as initiation of female sex hormone therapy. The Gender Dysphoria Trust International* offers further information and advice.

Sex-change surgery is not just physically traumatic, bringing permanent infertility and impotence, it can also cause considerable psychological and psychosexual trauma. However, by carefully integrating the man into his new sexual role, the risk of serious emotional disturbance can be reduced and many transsexuals find peace of mind for the first time in their lives once the transformation has been achieved.

Male menopause

Middle-aged men often complain of a variety of symptoms similar to those suffered by women going through the menopause. Men may not suffer from hot flushes and night sweats, but they certainly can experience many of the others, such as headaches, loss of memory, difficulty making decisions, lack of confidence, lethargy, exhaustion and depression. In contrast to menopausal women, men can retain their fertility well into old age; however, surveys show that middle-aged men notice a steady decline in their sex drive and are more likely to have difficulties getting and maintaining an erection, as a result of which their sexual performance can suffer.

Currently medical experts disagree as to whether this common phenomenon among men, popularly referred to as the mid-life crisis, is hormonal (like the female menopause) or purely psychological. The menopause in women is associated with a dramatic reduction in the production of the female sex hormone, oestrogen, by the ovaries. In men, there is a drop in the production of the male sex hormone, testosterone, by the testicles; but this tends to be only a gradual reduction and it usually starts much later in life, after the age of 60.

One possible explanation for the symptoms of male menopause in men in their 40s and 50s is that some factor stops testosterone working normally – even though the absolute level of testosterone may still be normal.

Testosterone replacement therapy

Clinical research has suggested that testosterone therapy may sometimes be effective at relieving symptoms of the male menopause, or viropause, as it has become known. About 400 men between the ages of 30 and 80 have received treatment with testosterone at one private clinic in London and a moderate to marked improvement was reported in more than 80 per cent.

Testosterone is initially prescribed in tablet or capsule form for the first few months. If this treatment is successful, pellets of testosterone may then be implanted into the buttock to produce a long-term benefit, lasting up to six months. Men who receive testosterone therapy have a thorough health check first and, because of the possible link between testosterone treatment and prostate cancer, various screening tests are carried out to exclude this particular disease.

However, until carefully controlled clinical trials are organised to confirm the true benefits of testosterone, male hormone replacement therapy is likely to remain highly controversial. Treatment can only be obtained privately and the bill, for screening tests, drugs and consultations, is likely to add up to several hundred pounds.

Psychological factors

The female menopause is universally accepted as being the result of oestrogen deficiency, but it is also recognised that various psychological factors may contribute to the symptoms. In middle-aged men, the mid-life crisis is thought by most doctors in the UK to be purely a reaction to stress and other emotional pressures, with no relationship to testosterone deficiency.

There is no easy answer for those trying to negotiate a smooth passage through middle age. However, there are a few measures that can protect your emotional health and help to prolong any long-standing relationship you are in:

● take positive steps to prevent stress overload at work and at home
● follow a regular exercise routine to help you stay in good physical shape
● work hard at keeping the romance and sparkle in your relationship; if you are having sexual difficulties with your partner, try to talk openly about them and do not put off seeking professional help

- make the effort to get involved in new challenges, both physical and intellectual
- try not to resent your partner if he or she is developing a new role or career, or seems to be more successful than you are.

Genital cosmetic surgery

A new penis-enlarging operation, called circumferential autologous penile engorgement (CAPE), involves the removal of about 30ml of fat from the centre of the abdominal wall through a suction tube; this fat is then injected in several different areas around the shaft of the penis, just underneath the skin.

As a result, the penis becomes more bulky, with an increase in circumference of several centimetres. Not only does the man get to show a bigger bulge in his swimming trunks, but by having the base of his penis widened it is claimed that he will be able to achieve greater stimulation of the nerve endings in the outer part of a woman's vagina during penetrative intercourse.

Over 700 American males have already undergone this operation, which is done under local anaesthetic, takes up to an hour to perform and costs the equivalent of £1,800. However, further surgery may be required to improve the cosmetic result as the penis is often left lumpy rather than uniformly podgy. The technique is still under investigation and its future availability in the UK remains uncertain.

Circumcision reversal

For men unhappy about having been circumcised as a child, there is now a non-surgical technique for restoring the foreskin which relies on constant, gentle stretching of the skin on the shaft of the penis over the glans (head of the penis). Although this tissue-expansion technique might sound bizarre, it is commonly used in other forms of plastic or reconstructive surgery and is based on the methods practised by members of certain tribes to stretch their lips or earlobes.

The main complaint from men who have been circumcised is that constant exposure of their glans results in its surface becoming tougher and a lot less sensitive. They also lose the additional sensation from contact between the glans and the foreskin as it slides back and forth during masturbation or intercourse.

While it is possible to replace the foreskin surgically using a skin graft, this stretching of the penile skin is attractive to some men because it is seen as being more natural and, done properly, it should not be painful. However, the procedure requires considerable dedication, taking as long as three years before the glans becomes fully covered, depending on the tightness of the original circumcision. Information is available from the Uncircumcising Information Resources Centre* in California.

CHAPTER **5**

FATHERHOOD – A SURVIVAL GUIDE

IT DOESN'T matter whether you have been planning to become a father for months or years or if the news that your partner is expecting has come as a complete shock, your reaction is bound to include a mixture of emotions, such as pride, excitement and anxiety. Having a baby with someone can dramatically change your life. It will certainly require some adjustments to your relationship, as there is now going to be another person around who needs love and attention from both of you. Yet, for many couples, the experience of parenthood adds more meaning and depth to their lives, despite all the additional worries and responsibilities.

Inevitably, some men worry whether they are really ready to be fathers. It is not only the financial implications of bringing up children – perhaps with the loss of one of the parents' income and all those extra expenses – that is worrying. Society now expects the father to do a lot more than just enjoy the fun that led to the conception and boast at work and in the pub about his children's achievements. This chapter is intended to help you through the minefield of modern fatherhood.

Health tips before conception

For couples planning to start a family, it is a good idea for both prospective parents to change to a more healthy lifestyle to reduce the risk of birth defects. A number of useful measures can also be taken by a man to improve the health of his sperm and thus increase the chance of his partner conceiving (see also infertility, *pages 138–9*). Remember that each sperm takes about ten weeks to develop and that it can be damaged at any time over this period.

Health tips

Stop smoking   A man who smokes tends to produce fewer sperm and have larger numbers of damaged sperm, which can impair his fertility. If a woman smokes while she is pregnant, she is more likely to go into premature labour, more likely to have complications during childbirth, and her baby's growth can be restricted. By giving up smoking together, couples have a much greater chance of the woman becoming pregnant and having a healthy child.

If either parent is still smoking, or starts again once the baby is born, there is an increased risk that the child will suffer from recurrent chest infections or asthma.

Cut down on alcohol   Regular heavy drinking may reduce the number of sperm produced, as well as damaging them, thereby lowering the chance of conception. Also, if a woman drinks heavily while she is pregnant, particularly in the first few weeks, she is more likely to miscarry or have a baby born with various abnormalities, including mental retardation. Cutting down on alcohol together will make it easier for your partner to succeed.

Eat a healthy diet   A lack of vitamins and minerals can interfere with sperm production and with the growth of a baby in the womb. Healthy eating habits are important throughout life, but particularly for your partner from the moment she becomes pregnant.

Exercise regularly   Your partner will find pregnancy and childbirth easier to cope with if she is physically fit to start with. If you exercise together, your health will benefit as well.

Practise relaxation   Couples who are stressed, particularly if the source of their worries is a failure to conceive as quickly as expected, often succeed in starting a family once they stop trying so hard and allow their love-making to be spontaneous and relaxed.

Keep your testicles cool   Anything that raises the temperature of your testicles can reduce sperm production: for example, being over-weight or wearing tight underpants or trousers. Wear cotton boxer shorts and, if you have a paunch, take steps to lose weight (*see pages 67–8*).

Sperm problems   Exposure to radiation and certain chemicals can impair fertility by damaging sperm. If these risks apply to your work, always follow safety guidelines.

If there is any inherited condition in your or your partner's family, such as sickle cell anaemia or Huntington's chorea, it is a good idea to receive genetic counselling before you start a family to establish the odds of your children being affected. Also, if any of your partner's relatives have been ill as young adults or developed a serious illness before the age of 50, you should try to find out whether an inherited disorder might have been responsible.

Men who are HIV-positive are usually discouraged from having children, because of the risk of the baby, as well as their partner, becoming infected with the virus. However, a new technique is being developed in Italy whereby HIV-infected cells are removed from ejaculated semen prior to the sample being artificially inseminated into the female partner.

Your partner's pregnancy

Being pregnant can cause a variety of minor complaints, such as back pain, indigestion, constipation and difficulty sleeping. Most women become irritable and very tired at times, particularly in the early and late stages of pregnancy, and your partner may want more attention paid to her and her needs than she did before she became pregnant.

To help you become more understanding and better prepared to make the necessary adjustments to your life while your partner is pregnant, it is a good idea to find out what pregnancy really involves in terms of the physical and emotional changes. Even if you are one of the few men who are unwilling or unable to attend the occasional antenatal class, you can still learn a great deal about pregnancy from the various good books that have been written on the subject.

Go with your partner when she has to attend the antenatal clinic, not necessarily to every appointment, but particularly at any time when there are specific worries or problems. That way you will be confirming to your partner that you are taking part in the pregnancy, showing interest and offering invaluable support. If there was a problem with the birth of a previous child, go together to talk to the staff who attended, or who are aware of the circumstances, so you can be reassured about what really happened and whether there are likely to be difficulties next time around.

Encourage your partner to discuss openly any anxieties she might have about the pregnancy and impending delivery. The more support you can give, the stronger your relationship will become. However, don't neglect to express your own fears and needs. You may even suffer a few pregnancy symptoms yourself, in sympathy, although any nausea, indigestion and difficulty sleeping are likely to be stress-related.

There are three main stages of pregnancy, known as trimesters, each stage three months long and characterised by specific changes in the mother and her baby:

First trimester

The embryo grows to about 5cm long and all its major organs develop. The mother will typically notice her breasts beginning to swell and they will often feel tender.

During this early stage of pregnancy, you must be prepared for your partner to complain of extreme tiredness at times and for her mood to vary suddenly from one day to the next. If your partner is suffering from morning sickness, you can help relieve this symptom by bringing her dry toast or biscuits, mineral water or weak tea first thing each morning.

You may also have to adjust your eating habits and, if you don't already do so, take a more active part in the cooking, as strong odours may aggravate your partner's nausea at all times, not just in the mornings.

Second trimester

This is often described as the blooming stage of pregnancy, because most women feel fit, healthy and full of energy at this time. Your partner may start to resent your attempts to offer help and support about the house, protesting about your apparent desire to treat her like an invalid, so be prepared to back off a little.

Women usually put on over half of their total pregnancy weight gain over these three months, with the baby growing rapidly and the uterus swelling upwards to cause the abdomen to distend. Your partner may have an increased appetite at this time, but she should not be eating for two. The actual increase in demand for food energy is only around 300 calories a day, so encourage your partner to fill herself up on high-nutrient, low-calorie snacks (see page 61).

Third trimester

During the final three months, many women again begin to feel tired as the delivery draws closer; now you should make even more effort to help out with everyday chores like shopping and ironing. Your partner may also start to worry about giving birth, so be prepared to talk through these worries.

A variety of complaints can develop, including breathlessness, swollen ankles, back pain, feeling faint and frequent need to pass urine. Getting comfortable in bed will also become more difficult, so find some extra pillows and cushions to support your partner in a more upright position.

Sex during pregnancy

Many women find that their sex drive is reduced during pregnancy. There are a number of possible reasons for this. First, your partner may be anxious about the changes in her body shape and feel that she is no longer attractive to you. It is therefore important to be tactful and reassuring, and to continue to demonstrate your physical attraction to her through kissing and cuddling, even when this is not going to lead to full intercourse.

Another barrier to sex may be the fear that penetration may injure the baby, introduce an infection, or lead to premature labour. Some women believe the myth that if they have an orgasm, this will in some way damage the baby.

There is certainly no evidence that sexual intercourse or orgasm can harm the baby and, as long as the man is not carrying any sexually transmitted disease, there should be no risk of infection to the mother or child. It has been suggested that sexual intercourse in late pregnancy with the man on top may occasionally hasten the onset of labour, sometimes by causing premature rupture of the membranes. However, this does not appear to happen with other sexual positions, which are usually more comfortable for her anyway.

Sex can normally continue throughout pregnancy, but remember your partner's breasts are likely to be tender during the first few weeks and, for the sake of comfort, you may have to use a side-to-side or rear-entry position in the third trimester. Circumstances in which sexual intercourse will have to cease include the onset of abdominal pain or vaginal bleeding at any stage of pregnancy, when medical advice should be sought. The doctor may advise a woman not to have sexual intercourse if she has a history of previous miscarriages or there is a continuing threat of premature labour.

Attending the birth

No man should feel obliged to attend the birth of his baby, although those fathers who have witnessed the event usually describe it as a rewarding experience and say they feel much closer to their baby as a result.

Often the man has a false perception about how much blood and suffering is actually involved and, once he has been reassured, he is likely to be far happier about being there. Of course, your partner may not actually want you there, in which case you should respect her wishes.

Having agreed to attend the birth, you should find out more about labour – either from books or by attending the antenatal classes – so you can provide useful support. Discuss the birth plan with your partner, so you are aware of her wishes regarding issues such as pain relief and holding the baby immediately it is born.

Make sure your partner knows how to contact you at all times from at least the 36th week of pregnancy onwards, and if you plan to drive her to the hospital have a trial run to check the route and timing.

In addition to providing emotional support and helping pass time in the early stages, you can assist your partner in labour in many other ways:

- you can act as a guide and interpreter – many women find it difficult to keep track of what is happening around them and don't take in everything that is being said
- you can provide extra nursing care, giving your partner regular sips of water, mopping her brow with a damp flannel, gently rubbing her abdomen during a contraction, massaging her back to ease discomfort and helping her change position
- you can remind her about her breathing and relaxation exercises, to relieve the tension of each contraction, and encourage her when the time comes to push.

The new baby

You should be prepared for your partner and new baby to come home within the first three days after the delivery. Over these first few days, a new mother will need a great deal of support. She is likely to feel uncomfortable, with bruising and possibly stitches from the birth and her nipples may be sore if she is breastfeeding. Even if the baby is being bottle-fed, the mother's breasts are bound to become tender and engorged with milk.

Your partner needs to be given as much opportunity as possible to rest and catch up with her sleep. Childbirth is an exhausting process and the new baby will initially be demanding a feed every few hours, day and night.

Certainly, it is a good idea to be at home with your new baby for the first week or so, not just to offer support, but also to allow you to get more involved and thus avoid feeling left out. Don't be surprised if you feel frightened about taking responsibility for your baby, even if it is only for an hour while your partner takes a nap. Although some antenatal classes do include lessons in how to hold a baby and how to do things like change nappies, bathe, dress and feed your baby before he or she actually arrives on the scene, a lot of these tasks will simply have to be learnt as you go along. If you watch your partner, you will soon pick up the basics and, in every minute you spend alone with your baby, you will learn more about his or her needs and become more confident.

Unfortunately, many fathers don't make the effort to get involved and, as a result, start to feel lonely, jealous and rejected. Rather than openly discussing his anxiety and anger, the father finds an escape by burying himself in work or spending more time out with friends. His partner, in turn, then becomes annoyed about his attitude and lack of support. To avoid this breakdown in communication, ask your partner what help she needs and make it known that you want to be shown how to do all the different tasks relating to the care of the baby.

One particularly important job for the father is to help out with the other children if this baby is not the first. There are bound to be some feelings of jealousy towards this intruder, which are understandable but need to be defused. Encourage your older children to get involved with the new baby, but don't force them. While the new baby is being showered with attention and gifts from all your family and friends, take time out to show your love and affection for the others and give them a treat or present; the mother should also spend time alone with her older children, leaving Dad to take care of the new baby.

Coping with a crying baby

All babies cry when they need something: it is the only way they can call out for help. Over the first two weeks of life, the average baby cries for up to two hours a day, which reduces to one hour a day after the age of three months. Your baby may cry more than this, even though he or she is perfectly healthy.

Every baby has a unique range of cries which you and your partner will soon learn to recognise, including a hunger cry, a wet nappy cry, a tired cry, a temper cry and a pain cry. You should start by going to your baby promptly each time to show that you are there when you are needed. Always handle the baby smoothly so he or she feels at ease in your arms.

Hunger is the usual reason for crying; a new baby may want milk every two hours at first. If a baby cries soon after a feed, this may be due to colic, in which case the baby will typically pull its legs up, scream and go red in the face. For colic, try rubbing your baby's tummy and gently bend and straighten its legs. A teaspoonful of gripe water or a colic remedy from the pharmacist containing activated dimethicone may also help.

Some babies need a lot of attention and cry because they are bored. Therefore, make sure your baby has a mobile or pictures to look at, or a toy to hold. A baby chair lets the baby watch what is going on, but don't put this chair anywhere unsafe or unsteady.

Alternatively, your baby might not like too much attention and may be easily startled. The best way to calm him or her is with cuddling and gentle rocking, talking or singing quietly, or playing music.

If your baby won't settle down to sleep, you can attempt to solve this problem in a number of ways:

- if you are working, don't come home and immediately start a lively game which gets your child over-excited. There should be a bedtime routine which calms your child down for the night. Even very young children enjoy a bedtime story
- if baby wakes in the night, give a feed, change the nappy if necessary, but don't have the main light on and don't play or make a lot of noise
- some babies settle more quickly if they are given a dummy to suck on, but don't dip this in milk or fruit juice or give your baby a drink

as a comforter as the sugar will rot the teeth, even before they have broken through

- make sure the baby's room is not too hot or cold and that the curtains shut out the light properly. You can warm the pram or cot with a hot water bottle, but take it out before putting the baby down

- wrap the covers firmly around to make your baby feel secure, but avoid overheating him or her by putting too much bedding on, and leave one arm free if your baby likes to suck his or her hand or fingers

- be prepared to allow your baby to cry for a few minutes; it is quite common for babies to cry as they are settling down to fall asleep

- if your child keeps calling out, go through the settling-down process again, but try not to take the baby out of the cot or pram unless you really have to

- the noise of a vacuum cleaner appears to get some babies off to sleep, but make sure it doesn't overheat if you have to leave it on

- a ride in the pram or car is another way to settle your baby, but it is not a good idea to make this a habit

- don't hesitate to take your baby into bed with you if that is the only way you are all going to get some sleep, unless of course you are under the influence of drink or drugs, in which case might you roll on top of him or her.

Controlling your temper

Parents whose baby won't stop crying may soon find that the love they have for their child turns to anger and frustration. The constant crying exhausts their patience and leaves them nervy and irritable.

First, it is important to realise that you can safely leave your baby crying. It won't cause any harm unless the baby has some medical problem, like a heart condition or a hernia. So put the baby out of earshot in another part of the house for a few minutes to give yourself the chance to unwind. If you are able to relax, this will help calm your baby when you return.

If you are afraid of losing control, find someone else you can trust to do the comforting and take your baby out. Don't be left alone with your baby if you can't cope with the crying. Call CRY-SIS★ if you need advice and support.

Any baby who seems to be crying excessively should be checked out by the health visitor or doctor. There may be a treatable cause, such as an allergy or infection.

Understanding the 'baby blues'

Giving birth and caring for a new baby are events that are emotionally as well as physically stressful. It is therefore hardly surprising that most women start to feel tired and tearful a few days after the delivery. Don't be surprised if your partner suddenly cries for no apparent reason, complains of feeling unable to cope, or says she is afraid she won't be able to take proper care of the baby. This is a common reaction to childbirth, which is popularly referred to as the 'baby blues'.

It is only when these feelings last longer than a couple of weeks, become severe enough to disrupt relationships in the home or begin to threaten the baby's welfare that a diagnosis of postnatal depression is made and treatment from a doctor is required.

To help your partner through the baby blues and reduce the risk of her becoming more severely depressed:

- get the house prepared before the baby's arrival
- make sure she has enough support over the first few weeks
- don't allow too many visitors at once
- ask for extra help from family and friends if you need it, for example, to babysit while you go out together
- encourage your partner to talk about her feelings
- suggest she joins a local parent and baby group.

The risk of postnatal depression is greater if there is some other source of stress, such as money worries or illness affecting the baby. Also, women who have suffered from depression before, even if it was unrelated to childbirth, are more likely to develop serious postnatal depression. However, there are some women who become depressed for months after having a baby, for which the only explanation is the hormonal changes that occur around this time.

If your partner is suffering from postnatal depression, the doctor will usually prescribe antidepressants and may also refer her for psychotherapy. Only a few extremely severe cases require admission to hospital to stop the mother harming herself or her baby.

Sex after childbirth

For at least the first two weeks, it will rarely be possible to resume normal sexual relations. Your partner will be far too sore owing to the bruising, scratches or small tears in the lining of her vagina and vulva, and she may have had stitches too. Also, sex would be messy because of the blood-stained discharge (lochia) that continues to drain from the uterus for some time after childbirth.

However, even if it is too soon to start having sex again, it is important to continue showing physical love and affection towards your partner with kisses and cuddles. Sex does not always have to include penetration or genital stimulation – there are other ways to make each other feel wanted and other erogenous zones on the body.

As the vagina and vulva heal, the soreness should soon ease off and the lochia will normally have cleared within a couple of weeks. Your partner may than decide she is ready to try sexual intercourse, but remember to take things slowly and gently at first.

About four in every ten women still feel uncomfortable six weeks after the delivery. This may be due to persistent bruising and inflammation, although sometimes the stitching may be a little tight. Also, some women notice they are dryer than they used to be due to a reduction in vaginal secretions, particularly if they are breastfeeding, as a result of the change in hormone levels this causes. Your doctor may recommend a lubricant, but make sure it is water-based, as oil-based lubricants may weaken a condom if that is the method of contraception you are using. Usually, all the discomfort during sex will have disappeared within three months; only a few women require some form of corrective surgery.

Because of the stretching of the tissues that occurs during a vaginal delivery, there will inevitably be loss of muscle tone in the vagina and some loss of sensation during intercourse as a result for both you and your partner. This may be more of a problem if stitches have been put in too loosely. Sensation should return to normal over the first few months, as the vaginal muscles regain their tone, helped by your partner remembering to do her pelvic floor muscle exercises regularly each day. Again, a few women may require corrective surgery.

Research into sexual behaviour has shown that one in three mothers are having sex again within six weeks of the birth and the majority have resumed sexual intercourse by three months. However, over half of these women reported that they initially had less interest in sex than before.

There are a number of reasons why women are less keen on sex after childbirth. First, it is important to appreciate just how tiring looking after a baby can be. At the end of the day, most new mothers just about have the energy to collapse into bed. Another common concern is the fear of falling pregnant again, so make sure you have agreed on a reliable method of contraception. Pregnancy can happen even before your partner has had her first normal period after the birth – don't believe the myth that she can't get pregnant while she is still breastfeeding.

Within a year most women start enjoying sex again as much as they did before the pregnancy. The key to preserving your love and affection for each other, despite any initial sexual difficulties, is to try to talk openly and honestly about these problems. You can't expect good sex if the rest of your relationship is not going smoothly. It takes a while to adjust to having a new member of the family and, if you are to stop a gap opening up between you and your partner, you need to make the time and the effort to discuss and resolve each new difficulty as it arises.

Be sensitive towards your partner's feelings about her own physical attractiveness, but encourage her to do all her postnatal exercises every day, especially those designed to strengthen her pelvic floor muscles. Don't expect her figure to return to normal at once: it may take many weeks for the muscles in her abdomen to become firm again. As a result of the breast changes that occur normally during pregnancy, her breasts may end up smaller and less firm than before.

The father's role

Children need to be able to relate to their father. Although he may be working hard to provide the necessary financial support for his partner and children, he must also spend 'quality time' at home to build a relationship with his family.

Children tend to see their father as a role model. They may not appear to take much notice of what he says to them, but they are strongly influenced by his behaviour and attitudes. How the father handles a particular problem sets an example to the child, affecting the way the child responds in a similar situation.

Children are constantly seeking to gain their father's approval and respect, which is why it is important to become involved in their achievements at school and at play. Unfortunately, there is a risk that parents will start to use a child's performance to satisfy their own previously unfulfilled ambitions, which may lead to their pushing the child too hard, or for the wrong reasons. If this starts to happen, both parents need to step back and remember that children deserve unconditional love and support, regardless of success or failure.

Parents of a child who has been having problems at school, for example, bullying, may not realise, through no fault of their own, that anything is wrong. There is no easy answer to this. You simply need to keep an eye and ear out for clues and create an atmosphere in your home in which your children feel they can approach you with their difficulties without worrying that they are letting you down by not being able to sort things out for themselves. However, it is not a good idea to pester children with questions. Simply give them the time and opportunity to speak out and then listen to what they have to say.

It is important that you and your partner are consistent in the way you discipline your children. If you do smack a child, it should not be for something trivial, not be hard enough to cause injury and not just be an outlet for your lack of patience or frustration. Any time you feel the urge to lash out, walk away to give yourself time to calm down.

Living with a teenager

Few teenagers pass through their adolescence without at least some emotional or psychological upset, as they struggle to find their own social identity and come to terms with new desires that they may initially be unable to fulfil during the difficult transition into adulthood.

Adolescents will often challenge the authority figures and symbols in their lives, just as a normal part of trying to establish their independence. To help them identify with their friends and give them a sense of belonging, adolescents also tend to adopt the extreme styles of behaviour and dress of that particular group.

Here are a few guidelines to help you and your partner survive these turbulent years:

- try not to be upset by arguments. Remember they are a normal part of growing up and try to argue only over important issues

171

- listen to what your son or daughter has to say and try to reach a compromise. Although teenagers will generally ignore and even resent your advice, however sensible and tactfully worded, as they grow up they will become more receptive
- show an interest in their friends and leisure activities, but also respect their privacy
- be prepared to discuss sex openly
- ignore their appearance if you can – most teenagers eventually tone down their dress and behaviour on their own initiative
- agree on a reasonable curfew time, with a later hour allowed when there is no school or college the next day
- talk through feelings of anxiety or depression. Short episodes of depression in an adolescent are common, but prolonged depression needs medical help
- be on the lookout for signs of anorexia nervosa, such as always missing out on meals and an obsession with losing weight, which is often accompanied by excessive exercising; bulimia, in which bingeing is followed by vomiting, is also becoming more common
- be alert to the warning signs of drug or alcohol abuse, such as alternating periods of sleepiness and hyperactivity, sudden mood swings, shivering and slurred speech, articles and money disappearing from the house, but don't make this accusation unless you are convinced your suspicions are correct. Try to discuss the issues and risks (*see pages 89–98*) rather than laying down the law.

CHAPTER 6

COMMON HEALTH PROBLEMS IN MEN

THIS chapter explains not only disorders which are unique to men, but also a large number of conditions common to both sexes which are either medically serious or simply aggravating or embarrassing. This is not, of course, an encyclopaedia of every conceivable health problem.

The list is arranged in alphabetical order.

Acne

Acne is an extremely common skin complaint among adolescents. Mild cases are characterised by spots, whiteheads and blackheads appearing on the face, with a fresh crop of spots emerging as the older ones heal. In more severe cases, acne spreads to the skin on the chest, back and sometimes even the buttocks.

The cause of acne is an excessive build-up of sebum – the waxy substance produced by glands adjacent to the hair follicles which keeps the skin lubricated. As a result of this build-up, the channel that drains sebum to the skin surface may become blocked, causing the nearby follicle to swell and inflame, forming an angry-looking spot.

While the spot remains covered it is called a whitehead; if it opens up, exposure of the sebum to oxygen causes chemical changes, the spot darkens as a result and is popularly referred to as a blackhead. Occasionally, one or more of these spots may expand under pressure to form a cyst or abscess.

A number of factors can trigger or aggravate acne, the most important of which is the sudden increase in the production of male sex hormones around the time of puberty. These hormones, which women produce in small amounts as well, stimulate the release of sebum in addition to their influence on sexual development. Accumulation of bacteria on the skin, high humidity, certain greasy cosmetics and a few prescription medicines can also play a part in this condition. However, acne is *not* caused by eating chocolate or fried food, masturbation or having dirty skin.

To minimise problems with acne:

- wash your face twice daily with a mild, unscented soap
- wash your hair frequently and keep it up off your forehead
- avoid any aftershave cream or lotion that might block the hair follicles
- do not pick or squeeze your spots
- ask your pharmacist to recommend an acne preparation: these can be very effective in mild cases.

See your doctor if:

- the above measures fail to help
- spots have appeared in places other than your face
- you have developed abscesses or cysts.

Your doctor may prescribe low doses of an antibiotic to reduce inflammation around the follicles and to kill off certain types of skin bacteria. A gel containing benzoyl peroxide is useful for unblocking the sebum channels, which it does by peeling off the outer layers of skin. Drainage of sebum can also be improved using a cream, gel or lotion derived from vitamin A, known as tretinoin.

This vitamin A drug is also available as isotretinoin capsules, which can be very effective at controlling severe acne and reducing the risk of the skin being left pitted or scarred. However, isotretinoin is a powerful drug that can only be prescribed by a skin specialist at present, and only with extreme caution because of the risk of liver damage.

Most sufferers grow out of acne in their early twenties and in those few cases where there is some residual scarring, a cosmetic medical procedure, such as gently shaving off the top layers of skin (dermabrasion), will usually help.

AIDS

See pages 120–2.

Angina

Angina (see also heart attack, *page 204*) is cramp of the heart muscle, causing a transient pain or tightness across the centre of the chest that sometimes spreads to the neck, jaw or arms. In some men, it may be a particular activity that brings on the pain, such as the exertion of climbing a flight of stairs, or eating a large meal. For others, angina may be provoked by stress, anger or extremes of temperature.

Descriptions of angina vary from a mild aching sensation to a heavy, crushing pain; sometimes the discomfort is mistaken for indigestion or heartburn. Other symptoms that often accompany an anginal attack include sweating, nausea, dizziness and difficulty in breathing.

Angina is caused by a lack of oxygen and nutrients reaching the heart muscle, usually because the coronary arteries which encircle and supply blood to the heart have become clogged up with fatty deposits – a condition known as atherosclerosis. This narrowing of the coronary arteries prevents the normal increase in blood flow that should occur when extra demands are placed on the heart, such as during exercise.

The risk of atherosclerosis increases with age, but there are a number of lifestyle factors which speed up the development of fatty deposits inside the arteries. These contributory factors include tobacco smoking, lack of exercise, excessive alcohol consumption and eating a lot of foods that contain large amounts of saturated fat and cholesterol.

Men may develop angina as early as their 30s or 40s, whereas women are protected from atherosclerosis by oestrogen until the menopause, when there is a sudden decline in the production of this female sex hormone.

To confirm a diagnosis of angina, the doctor will normally carry out an electrocardiogram (ECG), which is a recording of the electrical activity passing through the heart muscle.

Treatment of angina includes using drugs to widen the coronary arteries (nitrates, calcium channel blockers) and drugs which reduce the heart's demand for oxygen by slowing the heart rate (betablockers). Surgical procedures such as angioplasty (insertion of a catheter with an inflatable balloon tip into the narrowed arteries to flatten the fatty deposits) or bypass grafting (attachment of a blood vessel to redirect blood flow around the blockage) successfully relieve symptoms in many people.

Self-help measures for angina sufferers include:

- stopping smoking
- exercising regularly but only until the symptoms come on
- relaxation measures to reduce stress
- avoiding exercise on hot or very cold days, or soon after a meal
- losing excess weight to put less strain on the heart.

Anxiety

The main causes of anxiety in men, both young and old, are worries about health, money and unemployment. People who have been involved in some sort of serious accident or incident (being attacked, for example) may develop a form of anxiety known as post-traumatic stress disorder in which they continue to feel anxious long after the event and its implications are over.

While anxiety is a perfectly normal reaction to any problem or fear that cannot readily be resolved, it may become a disorder in its own right if it is so intense or prolonged that it prevents the individual from thinking clearly or rationally, sleeping properly, or coping with everyday activities.

Psychological symptoms related to anxiety may include difficulty concentrating, irritability, being easily distracted, getting tired easily but having trouble falling asleep at night, loss of appetite and a sense of impending doom. Some of the more common physical symptoms are palpitations, muscle tension, trembling, sweating and a feeling of suffocation. Mistaking these symptoms for a physical illness only serves to make the anxiety worse.

Self-help measures to relieve anxiety include:

- talking about the problem to a trusted friend, neighbour or relative who is a good listener and whose opinions you respect; sharing worries and feelings can put them into a calmer perspective
- talking to someone who has been through a similar experience, for example, by contacting the appropriate self-help group
- relaxation exercises, regular physical activities and meditation (*see* **Chapter 3**); if you know you tend to be anxious, try practising a relaxation technique regularly, not just when a crisis is already under way.

If symptoms of anxiety persist or recur despite these measures it is important to seek professional help. According to the Royal College of Psychiatrists, prolonged or severe anxiety is only rarely due to any significant mental illness, so there is no need to be scared of seeing a doctor. It is certainly better to receive treatment early, rather than late, and you are unlikely to be carted off to hospital against your will.

Your GP may decide to refer you for psychotherapy (*see Glossary*) to help you identify, understand and come to terms with the underlying reasons for the anxiety, which are often not immediately apparent. Treatment may last for several weeks or even months.

Tranquillisers can also be very effective as a short-term measure, but do not deal with the root cause of the anxiety and are not helpful in the long term because of the risk of addiction. Nowadays, doctors are advised to prescribe tranquillisers only for a brief period to help someone through an acute crisis. If they are taken regularly for longer than a couple of weeks there is a risk of addiction, with unpleasant withdrawal symptoms when the drug is stopped or the dose is reduced too quickly.

Asthma

Asthma is a lung disease characterised by recurrent attacks of breathlessness that are usually accompanied by wheezing, tightness in the chest and a cough. The individual finds it difficult to breathe in and even more difficult to breathe out. Attacks often occur at night or in the early hours of the morning. Children with asthma may not show any signs of wheezing but will usually cough, especially at night and also when they laugh or run around.

The cause of asthma is narrowing of the bronchi (airways) in the lungs, due to a tightening of the muscles in the walls of the bronchi (*see page 15*). There is also an increased production of mucus in the bronchi, which further interferes with the normal flow of air in and out of the lungs.

Asthma attacks can start at any age and may be brought on by a variety of different factors, including colds and 'flu, sudden strenuous exercise, breathing in cold air, an allergic reaction to pollen, mould, dust, feathers or fur, and stress or anxiety. For some people, however, there are no obvious causes that can be avoided.

To confirm the diagnosis, the doctor will usually arrange lung-function tests: for example, asking the individual to breathe out forcefully into a machine which measures the maximum air-flow speed. Sometimes this machine has to be taken home so that readings can be repeated at those times when the symptoms come on or worsen. Asthmatics have an abnormally low peak flow, particularly in the evening, in the early hours of the morning and during an attack.

Treatment of asthma consists of a bronchodilator, which relieves symptoms by widening the airways. Many asthma patients also receive additional medication (usually a steroid) which, by reducing inflammation, helps keep the disease under control, lowering the frequency and severity of attacks. Both the 'reliever' and the 'preventer' drugs are usually inhaled from a pressurised aerosol or a similar device.

Self-help measures for asthma sufferers include:

- never smoking; staying out of smoky atmospheres
- reducing exposure to dust mites by having someone else do regular vacuum-cleaning, dusting with a damp cloth, washing the curtains every few weeks, vacuum-cleaning the mattress and covering it with plastic, and using a mite-killing spray
- taking regular exercise, using the 'reliever' inhaler before starting
- asking your doctor for appropriate 'preventive' medication if your symptoms are interfering with your life by stopping normal activities or waking you at night
- having a 'flu jab every autumn.

See your doctor as soon as possible if your 'reliever' medication stops being effective or if you are having to use it more often. You should call for emergency help if you or the person you are caring for becomes severely breathless (for example, to the extent that it makes talking difficult), or if the skin becomes pale, clammy or turns blue. Most deaths from asthma are associated with a delay in calling the doctor.

Athlete's foot

Athlete's foot is an unsightly and irritating fungal infection that affects the skin of the feet. It usually starts between and underneath the toes, but can sometimes spread to the undersurface of the feet. Symptoms include itching and soreness of the skin, which may burn and then start to crack and peel. In some cases, the infected skin turns white, becomes inflamed and weepy, or begins to smell unpleasant.

The fungi which cause it – usually dermatophytes – feed off the protein-rich material (keratin) from the top layers of skin. Fungi are transferred from one person to another within the fragments of dead skin that are continually being shed from the feet.

Because the athlete's foot fungi prefer to grow in warm, moist surroundings, this condition is more likely to occur in people who don't dry properly between their toes. Two ways in which the infection may easily be picked up are when someone dries himself on a damp towel used by someone who already has athlete's foot, or by walking barefoot across a damp, contaminated floor, for example, in a communal shower, changing room or swimming pool.

Any man who uses communal bathing facilities regularly, such as swimmers and others who play sports, stands an increased chance of acquiring this infection, but it doesn't affect athletes alone: the fungi can be just as easily transferred in the family bathroom.

About ten per cent of the population are thought to be suffering from athlete's foot at any one time, although, for some unknown reason, some people seem to be resistant to this condition. Athlete's foot is more common in adults than in children and is usually picked up for the first time during the teen years. Men are more likely to develop athlete's foot, partly because of the closed, heavier shoes they wear, which encourage sweaty feet.

Self-help measures to combat athlete's foot include:

- drying the feet carefully, paying particular attention to the skin between the toes; using a separate foot towel helps prevent the fungi spreading to other parts of the body, such as the groin
- using your own towel and bath mat to protect other people who share your bathroom
- wearing socks made of natural materials (like cotton), rather than synthetics (such as nylon), which don't absorb sweat efficiently
- changing socks daily, and more often if you have sweaty feet
- wearing shoes with ventilation holes or a porous upper. Open-toe sandals are ideal but not practical for outdoor wear in wet or cold weather

- avoiding shoes which are a tight fit and which cramp your toes together
- not wearing the same pair of shoes on consecutive days: it can take at least 24 hours for them to air and dry out properly
- asking your pharmacist for an antifungal preparation and using it as instructed, which may be twice a day for four weeks or for at least ten days after the skin has cleared
- washing your hands after applying treatment to prevent the infection spreading to other areas of the body
- wearing protective shoes such as flip-flops in showers, changing rooms and around swimming pools.

See your doctor if the infection doesn't clear up or keeps coming back. You may need a more powerful antifungal drug that is available only on prescription. You should also seek medical help if the infection spreads to the nails, causing them to crumble or become discoloured.

Back pain

Back pain is the most common reason why people take sick leave from work. It is often accompanied by sciatica – pain radiating down the back of the thigh and leg – caused by irritation of one or more of the spinal nerves.

In the majority of cases, back pain is brought on by excessive strain on the lower spine, resulting, for example, from poor posture, being overweight, or doing a lot of heavy lifting and carrying. This strain may cause damage in the form of torn ligament or muscle fibres, displacement of some of the joints between adjacent vertebrae, or even a prolapsed disc, where part of the spongy material between two vertebrae is protruding and pressing on a nearby ligament or nerve.

Often an acute (sudden) episode of back pain clears up with bed rest and painrelievers before any investigations are carried out, so the exact cause may never be identified. However, if back pain is particularly severe or persists after 48 hours of taking painrelievers and lying flat, you should see a doctor. Immediate medical attention is essential if there are also symptoms of pressure on a spinal nerve, such as weakness, pins and needles, numbness or loss of bladder or bowel control.

Your doctor may prescribe strong painrelievers and muscle relaxants. Imaging of the spine may be done with X-rays, magnetic resonance imaging (an imaging technique using a powerful magnetic field and pulses of radiowaves) or CT scanning, where a detailed cross-section of the spine is produced using multi-angled X-ray beams under computerised control.

If there is only minor damage to the back, your doctor may recommend traction or manipulation, both of which can be extremely effective in relieving pain and muscle spasm in some cases. More serious conditions such as a stress fracture or a spondylolithesis (vertebra slipping forwards) may require surgery.

Other possible causes of back pain include osteoarthritis, ankylosing spondylitis (inflammation of vertebral joints), osteoporosis and, rarely, cancer.

Self-help measures to prevent or reduce back pain include:

- using a firm mattress, or placing a board under your mattress, to provide support at night
- losing excess weight to reduce load on the spine
- doing exercises to strengthen spinal and abdominal muscles, such as swimming
- using a heating pad or portable massager to relax muscle spasm
- wearing a lumbar support (helps some people)
- adopting the correct posture when sitting or lifting.

Sitting properly The chair should be adjusted to a height where your feet can be flat on the ground and knees level with or slightly above your hips. The seat should support three-quarters of the back of your thighs without digging in behind your knees. The work surface should be at elbow height.

Lifting safely Stand close to the object. Bend your knees, keep your back straight (but not uncomfortably so) and slowly rise, taking the load through your leg muscles.

Bad breath

Many people worry about having bad breath, but only a few actually suffer from this embarrassing problem. If you think your breath smells unpleasant, then pluck up the courage to ask someone close to you to sniff out the truth. Unfortunately, it is difficult to test your own breath, although occasionally you can tell by licking and then sniffing the back of your hand.

It is not uncommon to wake in the morning with a dry mouth accompanied by a stale odour. This is due to a reduction in the amount of saliva you produce while you are asleep, and tends to be worse if you breathe through your mouth, smoke, or drank a lot of alcohol the night before. A soft coating forms over the tongue and teeth and this begins to be broken down by bacteria in the mouth to release chemicals which smell foul. As soon as you clean your teeth, the coating and the odour should disappear.

If you follow a few simple measures you should be able to keep your breath fresh during the day. Eat regular meals, as chewing and swallowing boost your production of saliva, which acts as a natural mouthwash to clean and freshen your breath. Between meals you can use sugar-free chewing gum or mints, a piece of fresh fruit or a raw vegetable to stimulate the flow of saliva. Also make sure you drink enough fluids to keep your mouth moist.

Certain foods can produce a distinctive odour on your breath, which won't go away for several hours, whatever you do to try to mask the smell. Foods such as garlic and onions, once they have been digested, release sulphur-containing chemicals which get carried in the bloodstream to the lungs; the sulphur then gets breathed out over anyone who gets close.

The most common cause of persistent bad breath is poor oral hygiene. It is important therefore to clean your teeth at least twice a day, preferably after meals. Use a toothbrush that is in good condition, and check with your dentist that you are using the correct brushing technique. Failure to remove particles of food from around your teeth, especially meat, fish and dairy products, will allow them time to start decomposing with the release of foul-smelling chemicals. If you wear a denture, take it out before you go to bed; and keep it scrupulously clean by soaking it overnight, using a solution of sodium hypochlorite if it is made of acrylic, and chlorhexidine for metal.

Mouthwashes, freshener sprays and capsules are usually highly effective at masking bad breath. However, if you suffer from persistent bad breath, make an appointment to see your dentist; the usual reason is a rotten tooth or a gum infection that needs treatment. If your dentist is unable to find the cause, you should visit your doctor. Bad breath can sometimes be caused by a disease somewhere else in the body. Throat, sinus and lung infections, diabetes, kidney or liver disease, as well as certain medications, can all make your breath smell bad.

Body odour

Everyone has their own characteristic body odour. Most people have only a faint smell on their skin, which is often difficult to detect. Only when this smell becomes particularly strong or unpleasant should body odour be regarded as a problem. The fear of smelling offensive to others often drives many people to mask their natural smell, however mild it is.

Your body has roughly two million sweat glands and produces over three litres of sweat each day. Most of this sweat evaporates quickly. Hot weather, exercise and anxiety will cause you to sweat more and when it is humid the sweat won't evaporate as efficiently, making you feel sticky and uncomfortable. Some people produce large amounts of sweat, however cool, relaxed and rested they are. Overweight people tend to sweat a lot because they are more likely to overheat.

Fresh sweat does not normally produce any unpleasant odour unless you have been eating garlic, onions, curry or other spicy foods. It is stale sweat that has been on your body or on your clothing for several hours that smells. This is because the bacteria that normally live on the surface of your skin release chemicals from the sweat that give off a pungent odour. Sweat tends to build up in areas where it cannot evaporate easily, such as under the arms and in the groin. These areas also produce a special type of sweat which is more likely to go stale because it contains fats and proteins which encourage bacteria to grow, whereas sweat from other parts of the body is mainly salt water with only small amounts of waste products in it. The reason why sweaty feet often smell so bad is that the bacteria that rot sweat thrive in warm, airless places such as inside your socks.

Because body odour is usually due to the smell of stale sweat the best way to prevent it is to change your underpants and socks every day and to change your other clothes regularly. You should bathe or shower once a day and especially after exercise. But don't wash too obsessively as this can actually increase body odour by removing healthy skin bacteria. It is also important to dry properly as bacteria like living on moist skin. Some people find that applying talcum powder after a bath or shower helps keep their skin dry. If you tend to sweat a lot, wear comfortable, loose clothing and cotton rather than synthetics, so that your skin can breathe and the sweat can evaporate.

Using a scented talc to mask the smell of stale sweat may make the smell even worse. It is better to use a deodorant that contains an antiperspirant. Most antiperspirants work either by stopping bacteria from rotting the sweat or by preventing the sweat from evaporating, which then holds the smell in. If you decide to try a new brand, only use a little at first in case you are sensitive to it.

If you are worried about body odour, see your doctor. If you have a sweat problem, he or she may recommend you wash with antiseptic or antibacterial soap and may prescribe an antiperspirant which contains aluminium chloride. This works by reducing the amount of sweat you produce, but because it can irritate the skin it is usually applied only to non-sensitive areas.

In very severe cases an operation can be carried out to remove sweat glands from under the arms, but this often works for only a few months before the sweating returns.

Occasionally, body odour is caused by something other than stale sweat, such as fungal infection (e.g. athlete's foot) or an infected skin ulcer which needs special treatment. The smell may also be coming from somewhere other than the skin, for example, from bad breath due to tooth decay or gum disease, or from stale urine in an incontinent person.

Bronchitis

Bronchitis is a condition in which the main airways inside the lungs (bronchi) become inflamed (see page 15). As a result of this inflammation the normal production of mucus (also referred to as sputum or phlegm) is increased and it often becomes discoloured. The typical symptom is a loose cough which brings up yellow or green sputum.

An acute (sudden) attack of bronchitis is usually due to either a viral or bacterial infection of the airways. In most people it develops as a complication of a cold or 'flu, and other symptoms may include a fever, chest pains and breathlessness.

If you develop symptoms of acute bronchitis, see your doctor. You may be prescribed a course of antibiotics to deal with any bacterial infection present. Self-help measures include drinking plenty of fluids to help thin the mucus and an expectorant to make the sputum easier to cough up. But avoid cough suppressants such as codeine linctus as they will encourage a build up of mucus in the airways.

Using a steam vaporiser in your room, or inhaling steam, can help reduce congestion and make breathing feel easier, whereas spending time in a dry or smoky atmosphere will irritate the already sensitive airways, aggravating the cough as a result.

Sufferers from chronic (long-term) bronchitis have a productive cough on most days for three months or more every year. This is mainly a disease of smokers and those who have been exposed to high levels of air pollution. Apart from the persistent or recurrent cough, there may be wheezing, chest tightness and breathlessness on exertion.

Tobacco smoke and other air pollutants irritate the cells lining the bronchi, thereby increasing the production of thick, sticky mucus which clogs up these airways. When this irritation continues regularly over several years, there is a steady increase in the size and activity of the mucus-producing glands, which explains why the symptoms become prolonged and difficult to treat. Smoking also interferes with the normal process of clearing mucus, which is why smokers say they need a cigarette to help them cough to clear their lungs.

Stopping smoking and wearing a protective face mask in a polluted area can start to improve the condition at once. However, the longer the exposure has been going on, the more severe the damage is likely to be. Also, a chronic bronchitic becomes more susceptible to a bacterial infection which will cause his symptoms to flare up – doctors call this acute-on-chronic bronchitis.

Self-help measures for chronic bronchitis are as described above for acute attacks. Antibiotics may be prescribed when a flare-up of symptoms is due to an infection. The doctor may also prescribe a bronchodilator, usually as an inhaler, to try to open up the obstructed airways, but this drug won't work as well for chronic bronchitis as it does for asthma.

If you are susceptible to attacks of acute bronchitis, or you suffer from chronic bronchitis, you should visit your doctor at the first signs of a cold or of 'flu going to your chest. People with chronic bronchitis are also advised to be routinely vaccinated against influenza each autumn, as a dose of 'flu could make their chest condition a lot more serious.

Cancer

Cancer is not just one disease. There are many different types, each of which involves unrestrained growth of cells inside a specific organ or tissue in the body. The most common types of cancer in men are lung, skin, large bowel, prostate and testicular cancer. Stomach, pancreas and bladder cancers are also important causes of death in men.

By being aware of the warning symptoms of cancer, regularly examining your skin and testicles for abnormal changes and visiting your doctor for an urgent check-up if you notice any of the warning signals, the diagnosis can be confirmed at the earliest possible stage, which will give subsequent treatment a greater chance of success. Do not be afraid of being made to look a fool by seeming to panic unnecessarily. Even though the symptoms will often be due to a harmless or non-cancerous condition which will readily respond to treatment, in those few cases where the diagnosis does turn out to be cancer, any delay in treatment reduces the likelihood of a successful outcome.

In recent years there have been a number of advances in cancer treatment, with improvements in surgical and radiotherapy techniques and a wider variety of powerful anticancer drugs. Men who delay seeking medical help could be missing out on potentially life-saving therapies. .

Lung cancer

This is the commonest type of cancer in men by a long way, with over 100 new cases per 100,000 men diagnosed each year in the UK. The peak age for lung cancer is between 65 and 75 years; it is rare in men below the age of 40.

Cigarette smoking is the main cause of lung cancer. The more cigarettes smoked and the younger the age at which smoking started, the greater the risk. Cigar and pipe smokers have a lower chance of developing lung cancer, but their risk is still higher than for non-smokers.

Inhalation of tobacco smoke by non-smokers – known as passive smoking – has also been shown to be a risk factor for lung cancer. In addition, working with cancer-causing substances like asbestos may cause certain types of lung cancer, especially in smokers.

Symptoms may include a persistent cough, coughing up blood, breathlessness, chest pains and wheezing. The earlier the cancer is diagnosed, the greater the chance of a cure through surgery, radiotherapy and/or anticancer drugs. However, less than ten per cent of men survive for five years or more after lung cancer has been diagnosed, so prevention is crucial.

Skin cancer

In second place come the various types of skin cancer, the most common of which are squamous cell carcinoma, basal cell carcinoma and malignant melanoma. Taking all skin cancers together, just over 50 cases per 100,000 men are newly diagnosed in the UK each year. The most important risk factor for skin cancer is excessive exposure to sunlight.

With the exception of malignant melanoma, most skin cancers are no threat to life or health and can usually be cured if treated early. It is essential to report any changes in your skin – such as a new lump or bump, or an alteration in the shape, size or colour of a mole – to your doctor. Treatment is usually surgical removal, sometimes followed up by radiotherapy or chemotherapy.

Measures to reduce the risk of skin cancer are described in detail on pages 83–4.

Large bowel cancer

The third most common type of cancer in men affects the colon or rectum. Just under 50 new cases per 100,000 men are reported in the UK each year. This form of cancer usually develops between the ages of 50 and 70 years.

The exact cause of large bowel cancer is unknown, but genetic and dietary factors are believed to play an important part. Risk factors include eating a high-meat, high-fat, low-fibre diet and suffering from either ulcerative colitis or familial polyposis coli, an inherited disorder which causes hundreds of polyps (small growths) in the colon lining.

Symptoms of this particular cancer may include a prolonged change from your normal bowel habit, such as constipation or diarrhoea lasting more than ten days, blood mixed with stools and a sensation of not being able to empty your bowels completely.

Radiotherapy and, rarely, anticancer drugs may be used to treat large bowel cancer, in addition to surgical removal of the tumour. It may be necessary for the surgeon to create a temporary or even a permanent colostomy, where the cut end of the colon is brought to the surface of the skin and the faeces empty into a bag attached to the front of the abdomen.

About half of the people who have surgery for rectal cancer survive for at least three years after the operation and 40 per cent are alive ten years later. About half of the patients who are able to have a colon cancer removed surgically survive for five years or more.

Prostate cancer

Although the majority of men who develop prostate disease are suffering from benign prostate hyperplasia (see page 220), there are over 16,000 new cases of prostate cancer in the UK each year; the annual death rate from this disease is around 8,000. It occurs mainly in elderly men and although the exact cause is unknown, growth of the cancer is linked to the male sex hormone testosterone.

Pressure from a prostate cancer on the bladder and its outlet, the urethra, may cause difficulty with urination. However, for many men, when urinary symptoms are present they are due to a benign enlargement of the prostate, which is ten times more common than prostate cancer. Cancer of the prostate may not produce any symptoms until it has already spread to other parts of the body.

Screening for prostate cancer before it causes symptoms may be done by a rectal examination, whereby the doctor inserts a lubricated gloved finger into the rectum to feel whether the prostate is abnormally hard or knobbly. Other screening tests include an ultrasound scan and a blood test to measure the level of a particular protein (prostate specific antigen).

Because surgical removal of a cancerous prostate can lead to urinary incontinence and also impotence, the tumour may in many cases be left undisturbed. Radiotherapy and hormonal treatments are often used as an alternative, particularly when the cancer is already widespread when first diagnosed. Surgical castration may occasionally be carried out to slow down the progress of this disease.

The outcome depends on how early the cancer is diagnosed. As this type of tumour is relatively slow-growing, many elderly men die of another disease before the prostate cancer is life-threatening.

Testicular cancer

While cancer of one of the testicles is very rare before puberty and in old age, it is actually the most common cancer in men between the ages of 15 and 49 years. In 1992 an estimated 1,200 men developed testicular cancer; the lifetime risk of this cancer is 1 in 450.

The incidence of testicular cancer has doubled since the 1970s. Although the reasons for this increase are unknown, one possible factor is the greater number of young boys suffering from an undescended testicle, which has been found to make them five times more likely to develop testicular cancer in adulthood. Corrective surgery performed on an undescended testicle before the boy reaches the age of five makes it easier to detect any subsequent formation of testicular cancer.

There may also be a hereditary factor: for example, having a brother with testicular cancer increases this cancer risk by nearly ten times.

With one type of testicular cancer – a seminoma – radiotherapy is usually given routinely after surgical removal of the affected testicle. For the other main type – a teratoma – chemotherapy may be necessary if X-rays, an ultrasound scan or blood tests show any evidence of spread.

If picked up early, over 90 per cent of testicular cancers can be cured and, providing the remaining testicle is healthy, treatment should not interfere with fertility or potency. Regular self-examination of the testicles (*see page 83*) is therefore essential to allow early diagnosis. It does not need to be done obsessively, but men should be aware of how their testicles normally feel so that they can spot any change in size, shape or firmness.

Colds and 'flu

Colds and influenza ('flu) are viral infections which may cause a variety of familiar symptoms, including sore throat, fever, runny nose, sneezing, dry cough, aches and pains, weakness and swollen glands. The main difference between a cold and 'flu is that the latter typically makes you feel too ill to do anything other than stay in bed and lasts a few days longer. Also, if you are old or frail, 'flu is potentially fatal.

The viruses are spread through the air in tiny droplets of mucus or saliva when an infected person coughs, sneezes or speaks. Another common way to pick up the infection is rubbing your eyes with hands that have been contaminated with the virus (for example, from a door handle).

The reason why you can suffer one cold after another is that there are more than 100 different cold viruses. Acquiring immunity to one virus will not protect you from the next type of virus that comes along. You can try to keep away from anyone who is coughing and sneezing, but unfortunately people are contagious for up to two days before their symptoms actually appear.

With both colds and 'flu, you simply need to be patient while the infection runs its course. Although there are dozens of remedies to ease the symptoms (*see below*), there is still no cure. Antibiotics won't kill viruses, but they may be prescribed to treat or prevent any secondary bacterial infection such as sinusitis, bronchitis or pneumonia.

Most men with a cold or 'flu do not need to see their doctor. Useful self-help measures include:

- plenty of fluids to help replace water lost with the increase in sweating
- aspirin or paracetamol to take away aches and pains, and to bring down a high temperature (although aspirin should *not* be given to a child under 12 years old)
- salt water or aspirin gargles to relieve a sore throat
- warm drinks containing honey and lemon to ease a sore throat and dry cough
- inhalations and decongestants to relieve a blocked-up nose (do *not* take a decongestant by mouth if you have high blood pressure, heart disease or an overactive thyroid)
- using a vaporiser or humidifier to moisten dry air, which can otherwise aggravate a cough
- taking an expectorant for a loose cough, a suppressant for a persistent dry cough
- glucose (sugar) drinks to give you energy if you don't feel like eating.

Beware of taking more than one cold remedy at a time without checking with your pharmacist. Some may contain the same ingredients, so you could risk overdosing on a drug such as paracetamol, which might be fatal.

While you have a sore throat, fever or swollen glands, it is important to avoid taking any strenuous exercise, as this will not only make the infection worse, but could lead to a dangerous complication such as inflammation of the heart muscle (myocarditis). Also, after a bad bout of 'flu, rest for at least two weeks after the symptoms have gone to allow your body to make a full recovery.

See your doctor if you develop:

- a prolonged or high fever
- a cough producing coloured sputum or blood
- chest pains, facial pain or earache
- breathlessness or wheezing.

For most men, colds and 'flu are just a nuisance. However, if you are elderly or have any long-standing medical condition, particularly a heart or lung disorder, kidney disease, hormone abnormality, or any disease that requires you to take steroids or other immune system suppressants, there is a much greater risk of developing serious complications like pneumonia or heart failure.

An annual 'flu jab is therefore recommended for everyone in these high-risk categories. It is designed to provide immunity against the influenza viruses expected to be around that year. 'Flu vaccination is normally given in September or October. Do *not* wait until a 'flu epidemic has already started as the vaccine takes up to two weeks to become effective.

Dandruff

There is no need to be embarrassed if you suffer from dandruff. It is an extremely common problem which affects nearly half the population of the UK at some time in their lives. Dandruff is harmless and, most important of all, it is easy to treat.

The unsightly white flakes that appear in your hair and on the collar and shoulders of your clothes are actually clumps of dead skin cells which are being continuously shed from your scalp. Like the skin over the rest of your body, your scalp has a protective outer layer of dead cells which loosen and drop off, to be replaced by new cells moving up from the deeper layers. Normally, these skin scales are too small and too few to be noticed. It is when they clump together and start to flake off in much greater numbers that they become visible. Although excessive skin flaking can happen on any part of your body, it most commonly affects the scalp in the form of dandruff. If this condition does spread to other areas, usually the eyebrows, around the nose and the front of the chest, it is called seborrhoeic dermatitis.

Mild dandruff may be treated with a medicated shampoo bought from a pharmacist. This type of shampoo contains a substance which penetrates into the scalp and slows down the over-production of skin cells.

If your dandruff is accompanied by an itchy, inflamed rash on your scalp, make an appointment to see your doctor. You may need to be prescribed a corticosteroid cream or lotion to ease the inflammation.

In many cases, persistent dandruff and seborrhoeic dermatitis are the result of a yeast infection and the only effective remedy is an antifungal drug, prescribed as a shampoo for the scalp and a cream to apply to any other affected areas of your skin. Treatment normally has to be continued for at least one month and some people need to go on using the shampoo on a regular basis to stop the dandruff coming back.

Deafness

Deafness is perceived as a serious handicap because it acts as a barrier to normal conversation, encouraging the sufferer to become increasingly isolated and depressed as a result. In children, deafness can interfere with learning and speech development.

In conductive deafness there is something interfering with the normal transmission of sound waves through the ear canal, the middle ear and into the inner ear. Sensorineural deafness is caused by damage to the hearing mechanism in the inner ear, or to the acoustic nerve that carries sound impulses from the inner ear to the brain.

In adults, the most common reason for conductive deafness is a build-up of earwax; simply using eardrops and having the ear canals syringed with warm water by a doctor can restore hearing to a satisfactory level. A perforated eardrum can also result in conductive deafness; if this injury doesn't heal within two months, it may need to be repaired surgically. Another cause is otosclerosis, where one of the tiny connecting bones inside the middle ear – the stapes – becomes immobile. To correct this form of deafness, the rigid stapes bone is removed and an artificial replacement inserted.

Sensorineural deafness may be brought on as a result of prolonged exposure to loud noise, by a viral infection such as meningitis, or as a toxic reaction to certain medications.

If you are having trouble with your hearing, the first step is to overcome any embarrassment and discuss the problem with your doctor so that any treatable cause can be dealt with. Your GP may refer you to an ear, nose and throat (ENT) clinic or hearing-aid centre for a full assessment of your hearing and to see whether a hearing aid might help. However, be warned that in some parts of the UK there are long waiting lists for this service on the NHS. Also, however sophisticated the hearing aid, it will only be able to amplify those sound frequencies you have difficulty detecting; it will not give you perfect hearing.

A new treatment for complete sensorineural deafness that has only been available in recent years involves the insertion of a cochlear implant – an electronic device which can detect sound waves and transmit them to the brain. As a result of further refinements in the technology, a small number of people have had reasonable hearing restored with this device.

Depression

Everyone complains of being depressed occasionally, by which they mean feeling miserable, fed-up or pessimistic as a result of a disappointment or frustration in their life. Depression becomes an illness that needs medical attention or psychological treatment when it persists, deepens or starts to dominate an individual's existence.

This severe form of depression is typified by a loss of interest and enjoyment in life, feelings of helplessness or inadequacy and a lack of drive and motivation. The sufferer may start to have difficulty in making decisions and may no longer be able to cope at work; personal relationships with friends and family will be put under strain. He may begin to feel that life is no longer worth living.

About one in every nine men visits his family doctor because of a serious episode of depression. In some cases, there may be an obvious cause such as divorce or another relationship problem, unemployment, physical illness or money worries. However, depression hits others completely out of the blue, which makes it more difficult for their friends and family to be supportive. One common type of depression, known as seasonal affective disorder (*see pages 222–3*), is thought to be due to a chemical change in the brain brought on by a lack of exposure to ultraviolet light during the winter months.

Warning symptoms of a depression that should be treated if they persist include:

- insomnia and regular awakening in the early hours of the morning
- generalised aches and pains
- a sense of despair
- difficulty concentrating on one task
- a marked increase or decrease in appetite
- reduced sex drive
- loss of self-confidence
- crying for no apparent reason.

Confusion, agitation, extreme apathy and drinking more alcohol than usual can all be triggered by depression. Often a friend or relative has to persuade the depressed person to go to the doctor. Any threat of 'ending it all' should be taken seriously and the doctor called out if necessary.

A few people suffering from severe depression also occasionally feel elated and overactive at times. This condition is known as manic depression and is often treated with lithium.

A serious bout of depression should not be allowed to continue without treatment and will usually not disappear on its own. The risk of suicide is greatest among elderly men who have become isolated, or who are suffering from a long-term or painful illness, but the numbers of suicides in younger men is on the increase.

Treatment of depression, which is usually highly effective, may consist of:

- psychotherapy (*see Glossary*) or counselling from a trained professional who will encourage the depressed individual to talk about his feelings and to explore and confront the possible reasons for them
- antidepressants, which normally take a few weeks to lift the depression but can improve any associated anxiety or sleeping difficulties more rapidly. Unlike tranquillisers, antidepressants are not addictive. Treatment will invariably be continued for several months after the symptoms have gone to reduce the chance of a relapse
- electroconvulsive therapy (ECT), reserved for severe depression that is either not responding to other treatment or is accompanied by delusions. An electric current is passed through the brain for a split second with the patient under a light general anaesthetic.

SELF-HELP MEASURES TO TREAT OR PREVENT DEPRESSION

- talk problems and worries through with a friend or relative
- don't bottle up your emotions – it can help to re-live painful experiences and to cry if you want to
- take some form of regular physical activity
- eat a healthy, balanced diet even when you don't feel hungry
- don't drink alcohol to feel better – the immediate relief will only be followed by a deeper depression
- if the thought of retirement is at the root of your problem, make positive plans to stay mentally and physically active.

However, do not delay seeking medical advice if these measures do not help you.

Diabetes

Diabetes mellitus (sugar diabetes) is a common disorder of the body's metabolism caused by the pancreas gland either ceasing to produce, or producing very much less of the hormone insulin. Insulin is responsible for the absorption of glucose (sugar) from the bloodstream into the body cells, where it is converted into energy. Another important function of insulin is to control the uptake of glucose into the liver and muscle cells, where it is stored as glycogen (starch).

Symptoms occur partly due to an abnormally high concentration of glucose building up in the blood and partly to the body's inability to use or store glucose properly. Also, fat metabolism will be disrupted, resulting in an increase in blood cholesterol which in turn increases the risk of a heart attack or stroke.

There are two main types of diabetes: insulin-dependent, also known as juvenile-onset or Type 1 diabetes, and non-insulin-dependent, often referred to as mature-onset or Type 2. Insulin-dependent diabetes is the more severe form, which usually appears suddenly at some time before the age of 35. Destruction of the insulin-producing cells in the pancreas leads to complete or almost complete absence of insulin, which must be replaced by daily injections of an insulin substitute, either synthetic or from an animal. Cell destruction in the pancreas is thought to be due to an abnormal immune response to a viral infection or to some unknown environmental factor in those people who are genetically predisposed to this disease, but the cause is still under investigation.

In non-insulin-dependent diabetes, which usually comes on gradually after the age of 40, some insulin is still being produced but not enough to meet the body's needs. There is a strong genetic predisposition to this form of diabetes; however, ageing and obesity also play a key role in provoking its onset: as you get older, the pancreas begins to function less efficiently and excess body fat hinders the use of available insulin.

Whereas insulin-dependent diabetes usually causes obvious symptoms, many people with the non-insulin-dependent type only become aware of it as the result of a routine blood or urine test which reveals abnormally high levels of blood sugar, or the presence of sugar in the urine.

WARNING SYMPTOMS OF DIABETES

- blurred vision
- excessive thirst
- frequent urination
- fatigue and weakness
- numbness and tingling in the feet and hands.

The aim of treatment is to keep the blood glucose level as near normal as possible by keeping food and insulin intake well balanced. While insulin-dependent diabetics require insulin injections to achieve this, most non-insulin-dependent diabetics control their condition by means of a specific diet and/or antidiabetic tablets; the latter work either by stimulating the pancreas to produce more insulin or by making cells more sensitive to the action of insulin.

With proper treatment and monitoring, the risk of complications, such as damage to the eyes, nerves, blood vessels and kidneys, can be reduced and most diabetics are able to lead a full and active life.

SELF-HELP MEASURES TO ASSIST YOUR TREATMENT

- eat fewer refined carbohydrate (sugary) foods and more high-fibre, unrefined carbohydrate (starchy) foods, to avoid marked fluctuations in blood glucose levels
- cut down on fatty foods, particularly saturated fats
- lose any excess weight through regular exercise and the above diet

- get into a medication routine to reduce the chance of missing a dose
- carefully monitor either your blood or urine glucose
- have regular diabetic check-ups with a specialist in diabetes (this may be your GP or at a hospital clinic)
- carry or wear at all times a card identifying you as a diabetic in the event of an emergency
- be aware of the warning symptoms of hypoglycaemia (a dangerously low blood sugar level), which include feeling dizzy or drowsy, sweating, tingling, cold clammy skin, palpitations and headache. If such symptoms occur, a sugary drink or food should be taken at once to prevent collapse and coma.
- be aware also of the symptoms of hyperglycaemia (acetone odour on the breath, drowsiness, confusion and, in severe cases, lapsing into a coma), in which the blood sugar level becomes dangerously high. This may be caused by eating too many sugary foods and/or not taking enough medication.

Eye and vision problems

The most common reason for someone's vision becoming blurred is a problem with the focusing mechanism in the eyes. In young men, this is usually due to myopia (short-sightedness), a condition in which the eyeball has grown too long from the front to the back. As a result, light rays from objects in the distance are focused by the cornea and lens in front of rather than directly on to the retina. While close vision remains unaffected, anything more than a few yards away will no longer appear sharply defined: for example, there may be difficulty in recognising people at a distance.

For most men, myopia comes on so slowly that it is not picked up until a man has a routine eye test (*see page 85*). An optician can then correct the defect with spectacles or contact lenses.

In a man over the age of 45, his near vision is most likely to fail due to the common eye disorder presbyobia. A weakness develops in the muscles that change the shape of the lens in each eye. As a result, it becomes more difficult for the man to focus on small print and close objects. A man who has been wearing spectacles for short-sightedness will typically find that he has to take them off when he tries to read something.

To correct presbyopia, the optician can prescribe spectacles which, if the man is also short-sighted, can be fitted with bifocal lenses – one half designed for near vision, the other for distance vision. Because the focusing power of the eye characteristically continues to weaken as a normal part of ageing, stronger lenses may be required every year or two until all the focusing is being done by the spectacles; wearing spectacles will not itself make the eye muscles weaker.

Another common focusing problem is hypermetropia (far-sightedness). In this case, because the eyeball is too short, the light rays tend to be focused behind the retina. In young men, the muscles that change the shape of the lens to boost focusing power can usually compensate for this underlying abnormality. However, as the lens muscles weaken with age, hypermetropia may start to cause blurring of close objects and affect distance vision in more severe cases. Spectacles or contact lenses of the correct strength should immediately restore clear vision.

In astigmatism, the front surface of the eye loses its smooth, even curve and magnification in one plane is not the same as in another. Most people's eyes have a minor degree of astigmatism which does not need to be corrected with spectacles or contact lenses.

Any disturbance in your vision should always be checked out by an optician or doctor. Many different disorders can interfere with normal vision: most involve a particular structure in one or both eyes, but a few are the result of interference to the passage of nerve impulses from the retina to the brain, or damage to the area of the brain where pictures are received and interpreted.

Common eye disorders not corrected with lenses
Cataract
A cataract is a loss of transparency in the lens of one or both eyes, causing vision to become increasingly blurred, with red, orange and yellow colours becoming more pronounced than others. The risk of developing a cataract increases with age; in young men, there is usually a specific reason for this change: diabetes or a serious eye injury, for example. Surgical removal of the opaque lens and replacement with a tiny artificial lens implant usually restores normal vision.

Glaucoma
Glaucoma, in which abnormally high pressure inside one or both eyes interferes with the blood supply to the nerve at the back of the affected

eye(s), may cause permanent blindness. In some cases there are obvious symptoms – a painful red eye with blurred vision, or seeing coloured haloes around lights, for example. However, it is often only picked up during a routine eye examination if an optician or doctor carries out a pressure test. Because glaucoma runs in families, anyone who has a close relative with this disorder needs regular screening after the age of 40.

Treatment of glaucoma is with daily application of pressure-reducing eye drops and, sometimes, drainage surgery. Vision cannot be restored, but further deterioration can be prevented.

Retinal detachment
Separation of the retina from the outer layers at the back of the eye sometimes follows a blow to the eye, but, more usually, occurs spontaneously due to natural degeneration. Detachment is more common in men who are extremely short-sighted.

A retinal detachment may develop without any warning symptoms, with the man suddenly noticing a 'black curtain', which has obscured his vision in the affected eye. However, there will often be a burst of flashing lights as the tear stimulates the light-sensitive nerve cells in the retina, accompanied by the appearance of spots in front of the eye.

Surgical treatment of a retinal detachment usually achieves excellent results, as long as the operation is performed before the damage has spread to the central part of the retina (macula), an area densely packed with light receptors, which assists the perception of fine detail.

Glandular fever

Glandular fever, also known as infectious mononucleosis, is a viral infection which most commonly affects adolescents and young adults. It is sometimes called 'the kissing disease' because the virus may be carried in saliva exchanged during a wet mouth-to-mouth kiss.

Routine blood testing suggests that as many as 50 per cent of the population in the UK may have been infected with this virus. Only a small number of these people will actually develop symptoms, but all of them will continue to release the active virus into their saliva intermittently for the rest of their lives. Infection with glandular fever is most likely to be picked up from close contact with one of these symptom-free carriers, rather than someone who is obviously ill.

Typically, glandular fever starts with 'flu-like symptoms - sore throat, high temperature, headache, weakness, aches and pain - and soon afterwards lymph nodes in the neck, armpits and groin become swollen and tender. A blood test which shows the presence of abnormal antibodies in the circulation will confirm the diagnosis. However, some people suffering from a glandular fever-like illness have a negative blood test at first that only becomes positive after a few weeks.

Because it is caused by a virus, antibiotics will not cure glandular fever. The only treatment is rest and relaxation while the infection runs its own course. Trying to do too much too soon will increase the chance of a relapse. Glandular fever is not usually a dangerous infection, but it can be extremely debilitating and may last for many months. The individual may suffer recurrent episodes of relapse, during which he or she will be unable to cope with vigorous physical or mental activity.

One possible complication is liver inflammation (hepatitis) resulting in jaundice. In most cases, normal liver function returns within a few months.

Gout

Gout is a type of arthritis that characteristically attacks one joint at a time. The joint at the base of the big toe is the one most often affected. It develops when uric acid crystals are deposited inside a joint, which causes the affected tissues to become temporarily inflamed. During an attack, the joint becomes extremely painful and swollen, with redness of the overlying skin. Occasionally, uric acid crystallises as white deposits under the skin (tophi), which may then ulcerate and have to be removed surgically.

Men are ten times more likely to suffer from attacks of gout than women, possibly due to their higher consumption of alcohol, particularly beer, and possibly due to differences in protein metabolism. These attacks may begin any time after puberty in men, while women usually develop this condition only after the menopause.

Attacks may be treated with large doses of an anti-inflammatory drug and sometimes with the drug colchicine to suppress the inflammation rapidly. If the cause is abnormally high levels of uric acid in the blood and attacks are recurrent, the doctor may prescribe a drug which reduces the production of uric acid in the body, or a drug to increase the amount of uric acid passed in the urine.

Gout sufferers are advised to reduce their dietary intake of purine, which is converted in the body to uric acid. Foods to avoid because they are high in purine include organ meats (liver, kidney, heart), wild game, anchovies, mackerel, herring, scallops, sardines, whitebait and mussels. Foods to eat in moderation because they contain a fair amount of purine include other meats, poultry, fish not mentioned above, peas, green beans, lentils, spinach, mushrooms, asparagus and cauliflower.

Hair loss

There is no need to be alarmed when you find hairs caught in your brush or comb, or blocking the plughole after you wash your hair or take a shower. Everyone loses on average between 50 and 150 hairs each day. However, for each hair that drops out, a new hair from the same follicle normally grows up to replace it within three months.

The hair that drops out is in the resting phase of its growth cycle. At any one time around 10 per cent of scalp hair is in this resting phase, while the remaining 90 per cent is actively growing. Loss of hair is only considered to be a problem when it starts to produce bald patches and, even then, for most men baldness results from their genetic make-up rather than from any scalp or hair disease.

Hair loss in men is most commonly due to the hereditary condition known as male-pattern baldness, in which the hair first starts to thin out over the temples and crown to cause a receding hair line. Normal hair at these sites is replaced by fine, downy hair which eventually disappears altogether to create a slowly expanding bald area.

A few men who complain of going bald have developed one or more small, circular areas of baldness, where the exposed scalp looks and feels perfectly healthy. This condition, known as alopecia areata, remains a mystery to doctors. The cause is unknown and there is no consistently reliable treatment as yet, although, fortunately, the hair usually grows back within a few months.

Another common reason for bald patches is mistreating hair, for example, by brushing or combing it over-enthusiastically, pulling on it as a nervous habit, or adopting a hairstyle where the roots are under constant tension, for example, by pulling it into too tight a ponytail. It is also best always to use a soft-bristled brush to reduce the amount of trauma to your hair roots.

Occasionally, bald patches are due to a fungal infection, or some other skin disease affecting the scalp. In this case, the scalp will look unhealthy, there will usually be stubble rather than smooth skin and your doctor should be able to return your hair to normal by treating your scalp problem with, for example, an antifungal drug.

Factors which can cause sudden generalised loss of hair include severe stress, prolonged illness, a major operation, a crash diet and exposure to radiation. Once the individual starts to make a recovery, the hair will normally regrow within a few months. Temporary baldness may also be brought on by a number of popular medications including certain betablocker drugs, arthritis drugs and some of the drugs used to lower blood cholesterol.

There is also a rare inherited condition which, in addition to causing total baldness, results in a complete loss of body hair so that even the eyebrows and eyelashes disappear.

Whereas in the past, 'treatment' of baldness consisted of being fitted with a wig or toupée, nowadays a number of other measures are available. A hair-restoring solution has been developed from the drug minoxidil, which can halt the progression of hair loss and stimulate some hair regrowth. However, it only seems to help some of the men who suffer from male-pattern baldness and the hair that grows back tends to look rather fluffy. Stopping minoxidil leads to a gradual loss of any hair that has been gained within four to six months and so treatment has to be continued indefinitely. At present, minoxidil is only obtainable on a private prescription and one month's supply costs about £30.

A much more expensive option which is sometimes successful in covering up a bald patch is a hair transplant. Many factors influence whether such a procedure would work well, for example, the pattern and extent of hair loss, the texture of the hair and how curvy or wavy it is. Plugs or strips of skin are transferred from hair-bearing scalp to slits or holes made in a bald or thinning area and held in position under pressure. Sometimes, a small flap of scalp is removed as a separate procedure prior to transplantation to reduce the area needing a hair graft.

Hair transplantation usually takes three to four sessions, with four months between each, at a cost of several thousand pounds. The procedure is not available on the NHS. It is important to be patient after a hair transplant as grafted hair is usually shed, taking several months to start growing again and growing only very slowly at first. To avoid this problem of hair fallout and delayed regrowth, it is occasionally possible to cut a flap of scalp hair which is then repositioned across a cut section of bald scalp, leaving the blood supply to the graft intact.

Hair weaving and fusion techniques have also advanced considerably over recent years. However, even the more expensive synthetic hairpieces only last for about three years.

To cope with hair loss:

- try thickening shampoos and conditioners, which either coat the hair shafts or swell individual hairs. They can help conceal an area of thinning, but there is no shampoo or over-the-counter remedy that reverses baldness
- pat rather than rub your hair dry
- while your hair is still damp, try a different parting to give it more lift
- use a spray, mousse or gel to make your hair look fuller; however, overuse of these products may cause hair to become brittle, encouraging further hair loss
- avoid long hair at the back and sides if you are thinning on top as this will highlight the bald area by pulling hair away from it
- consider having a gentle perm to disguise thinning hair by making it lift and appear fuller
- if you wear a wig or hairpiece, ask your hairdresser to style it to create a more natural look.

Hay fever

Hay fever is an allergic reaction to pollen from trees, grasses or weeds, or to spores released from fungi or moulds. Symptoms of hay fever include sneezing, a runny nose, itchy watering eyes and occasionally wheezing. The proper medical name for this condition is seasonal allergic rhinitis.

Self-help measures to prevent or reduce the symptoms of hay fever include:

- staying indoors in the early morning (before 10am) when pollen counts are usually at their highest
- having the grass around your home mown regularly by someone other than yourself
- wearing a protective mask if you have to go outdoors when pollen levels are high

- keeping windows closed, particularly at night
- driving an air-conditioned car so that you can keep the windows and vents to the outside shut
- using a tumble dryer: pollen collects on clothes hung outdoors to dry
- asking your pharmacist to recommend an antihistamine medication, preferably one that doesn't cause dizziness or drowsiness.

See a doctor if your symptoms are severe or are making your life miserable. You should also seek medical help if you develop symptoms of allergic asthma such as a dry cough, wheezing or breathlessness. In addition to an antihistamine drug, you may be prescribed eye drops, a nasal spray, or an inhaler to widen your airways. A course of desensitisation injections may be successful in those people who are allergic to just one or two particular substances.

Heart attack

A heart attack, also known as a coronary thrombosis or myocardial infarction, is a serious condition in which part of the heart muscle dies. It occurs as the result of a blockage in the blood supply that provides the heart muscle with essential oxygen and nutrients.

In most cases, a heart attack is caused by the formation of a blood clot in one of the coronary arteries which encircle the heart. The clot characteristically develops in a section of the artery that is already narrowed by fatty deposits, a condition known as atherosclerosis. Less commonly, temporary spasm in the muscle wall of a coronary artery causes the obstruction.

There are about 160,000 deaths each year in the UK from heart attacks, making this by far the most common cause of death. Roughly one man in 12 will die of a heart attack before he reaches retirement age. Risk factors for a heart attack are divided into those you can and those you cannot do something about.

Unavoidable risk factors include being male, getting older, a family history of heart attacks and abnormally high blood cholesterol, or suffering from diabetes or high blood pressure. Avoidable risk factors are smoking, drinking too much alcohol, not taking enough exercise, being overweight and eating a diet rich in saturated fat, cholesterol and sugary foods.

Symptoms of a heart attack may include pain across the centre of the chest – typically a severe crushing discomfort lasting for at least 20 minutes – pain spreading into the neck, jaw, shoulders or arms, sweating, nausea, vomiting, palpitations, dizziness and breathlessness.

Anyone suspected of having a heart attack should be seen by a doctor as soon as possible. Most heart attack deaths occur in the first few minutes and could have been prevented if the appropriate first-aid measures had been carried out. It is therefore important to learn life-saving techniques, such as artificial ventilation and external cardiac compression, from a professional instructor, in case you have to help a heart attack victim whose breathing and heartbeat have stopped. A delay of even a few minutes while waiting for medical assistance is likely to prove fatal.

A new type of medication is now available which, injected into the circulation, can quickly dissolve the blood clots that cause most heart attacks. These 'clot-busting' drugs, such as streptokinase, can halt a heart attack and minimise heart muscle damage as long as they are injected within a few hours of the onset of symptoms.

In addition, painrelieving drugs will be given as well as drugs to treat any of the complications that may develop in more serious cases, such as heart failure or an irregular heartbeat. Surgical treatment of the blockage, following a heart attack, may include balloon angioplasty or coronary artery bypass grafting (see angina, *pages 175–6*).

To assist recovery after a heart attack, ask your doctor for clear guidelines on returning to normal activities, including sex. As a general rule, sexual intercourse can be resumed once you can comfortably climb two flights of stairs. Doctors now encourage heart attack patients to follow a graded exercise programme, assuming there are not medical factors that make this too risky. Regular physical activity after a heart attack has been shown to reduce the chance of a recurrence.

Heartburn

Heartburn is an extremely common symptom. This painful burning sensation under your breastbone can vary from a niggling discomfort to a pain so intense it may be mistaken for a heart attack. Often heartburn sufferers also complain of belching and a bloated feeling because they subconsciously swallow air in an attempt to relieve their discomfort.

Some men develop heartburn as a reaction to a particular food: for example, rich, fatty or spicy meals are often to blame, as well as acidic fruits and vegetables, like grapefruit and tomatoes.

Recurrent episodes of heartburn may also be caused by regurgitation of stomach acids into the oesophagus (gullet). A backflow of stomach acids can occur when the muscular valve which prevents this acid reflux is put under too much pressure as a result of, for example, overeating or being overweight. Carbonated drinks such as sparkling mineral water may bring on heartburn by raising pressure inside the stomach; coffee, smoking and alcohol may all provoke acid reflux by relaxing the valve.

Another cause for the valve not closing properly is a hiatus hernia, a common condition in which part of the stomach protrudes upwards into the chest cavity through a weakness in the diaphragm.

Typically, heartburn comes on within one hour of eating when stomach acid production peaks to aid digestion. Bending forwards, lying down and exercising too soon after a meal can also bring on an attack.

To help prevent heartburn:

- eat several small meals a day, and don't eat just before going to bed
- try to identify and avoid foods that bring on the pain
- cut down on alcohol, particularly neat spirits, and stop smoking
- don't bend over, lie down or exercise within one hour of eating
- try to lose any excess weight
- don't wear a tight belt or other restrictive clothing
- sleep with extra pillows, or elevate the bed head using 15-cm blocks
- take an antacid immediately after a meal.

See your doctor if you are suffering from persistent or recurrent heartburn and these measures have not worked. You may be prescribed a drug to reduce the amount of acid produced in the stomach, or a drug that tightens the muscular valve. In severe cases, surgery may be needed to strengthen the valve or repair a hiatus hernia.

Heart failure

This is a potentially serious condition in which the heart muscle is no longer able to pump efficiently. Although heart failure only rarely occurs in men under the age of 65, about five per cent of men in their 70s and ten per cent of men over the age of 80 are affected.

Failure of the heart muscle to pump is often the result of direct damage to the muscle fibres, following a heart attack or due to long-standing high blood pressure, for example. Other possible causes include a heart-valve defect, irregular heartbeat or excessive stimulation of the heart due to an overactive thyroid gland. Any lung disease which impedes the flow of blood, such as bronchitis or emphysema, can also lead to heart failure by putting extra strain on the muscle wall of the right ventricle.

Initially, the heart may compensate for its decreased pumping ability through activation of the sympathetic nervous system (*see pages 27–8*), along with the release of the hormone renin, which in turn stimulates the production of a substance known as angiotensin II, which constricts the blood vessels. However, these changes are usually unable to maintain normal blood flow indefinitely and start to contribute themselves to a further deterioration in heart function.

Symptoms of heart failure typically include breathlessness, made worse by exertion or lying flat, muscle fatigue, swelling of the ankles and, sometimes, abdominal discomfort due to engorgement of the liver. In addition to carrying out a physical examination, the doctor may confirm the diagnosis by arranging a chest X-ray, electrocardiogram (*see Glossary*) and an echocardiogram (ultrasound scan of the heart).

Drugs commonly used to treat heart failure include diuretics (which reduce fluid retention by increasing the volume of urine passed each day), an ACE inhibitor (which reduces the production of angiotensin II, improves blood flow and partially restores heart muscle function), digoxin (which stimulates the heart muscle to strengthen the power of its contractions) and a vasodilator (which eases the heart's workload by widening blood vessels around the body).

Finally, there are a number of self-help measures which may be recommended for someone who is suffering from heart failure, such as:

- raising the head of the bed to assist breathing
- gently exercising to improve heart and circulation function
- reducing salt consumption, which may otherwise encourage fluid retention
- elevating the feet when sitting to reduce ankle swelling
- losing excess weight to reduce strain on the heart.

Hernia

An abdominal hernia is the abnormal protrusion of an internal organ, usually part of the intestine, or fat, through a weakness in the abdominal muscle wall. This type of hernia is most common in older men, whose abdominal muscles tend to lose some of their strength and tone, partly due to their being less active and partly the result of putting on weight around the abdomen later in life.

If you notice a bulge in your abdominal wall, groin or scrotum see your doctor. The main risk from an abdominal hernia is obstruction of the intestine or its blood supply due to the protruding loop becoming compressed, which in turn can lead to potentially fatal complications.

Surgical repair is recommended in most cases to prevent complications occurring in the future. The operation is usually relatively easy for the surgeon to perform, taking about half an hour to complete and only keeping you in hospital for a few days at the most. Before returning to normal activities, particularly those which involve carrying or lifting, it is essential to follow a supervised programme of exercises to stretch and strengthen the abdominal muscles – otherwise, the risk of recurrence is much greater.

For those men who are not fit enough to have an operation, a surgical truss or corset may be provided to prevent the hernia from bulging through the muscle wall. For this to be effective, it must be possible to gently ease the hernia back inside the abdomen; the truss should be put on before getting out of bed and then worn all day.

If a hernia suddenly becomes painful, tender, swollen or inflamed, seek medical attention at once as these are signs that the intestine is under pressure.

High blood pressure

Everyone has blood pressure: this is the force that pushes blood through your arteries generated by the pumping action of the heart. The measurement of blood pressure comes as two figures: the higher reading is recorded at the moment the heart beats and the lower reading between beats when the heart muscle is relaxed.

Blood pressure varies throughout the day, increasing as a result of stress, exercise or pain and decreasing during periods of rest and relaxation. In a group of men, blood pressure measurements taken at rest will differ between individuals in the same way that their height and weight differ. The definition of high blood pressure is a reading above the accepted normal range, which according to the World Health Organisation is 160/95.

Before a diagnosis of high blood pressure is made, usually a resting value of greater than 160/95 must have been recorded on at least three occasions. Healthy young men would normally have a blood pressure well below this threshold, with an average reading of 120/80. But about seven per cent of men between the ages of 40 and 49 have a blood pressure greater than 160/95. Older men are more likely to develop high blood pressure because their arteries have become less elastic and narrowed by deposits of fat (atherosclerosis).

High blood pressure almost always develops without any underlying medical cause, although in a few cases the blood pressure has been pushed up by a kidney, blood vessel or hormonal disorder. Certain medicines, such as anti-inflammatory drugs, can also increase your blood pressure. The medical term for high blood pressure is hypertension, but tension (stress) is only one possible contributory factor.

Most people with high blood pressure feel perfectly well and don't have any symptoms. The condition is usually only discovered during a routine test. Occasionally, high blood pressure causes headaches, dizziness, nausea or blurred vision, but these symptoms usually have some other explanation.

Because untreated high blood pressure can result in a number of serious complications, you should have your blood pressure routinely checked by your GP or practice nurse at least every five years and annually over the age of 55. These complications include thickening of the heart muscle and damage to arteries, particularly in the heart, brain, kidneys and eyes, thereby increasing the risk of heart failure, heart attack, stroke, kidney failure and loss of vision due to haemorrhage in the retina at the back of the eye.

Not everyone with high blood pressure needs drug treatment. Measures to help correct high blood pressure include losing excess weight, taking regular exercise, eating a high-fibre, low-fat diet, cutting down on salt, restricting alcohol intake and stopping smoking. Relaxation and meditation can also help. Avoid activities that cause a prolonged build-up of tension in the muscles, such as heavy lifting and powerful gripping, as these can lead to a big increase in blood pressure. If blood pressure remains high despite these measures, there are several different antihypertensive drugs your doctor can choose from.

Insomnia

People vary a great deal in the amount of sleep they need to wake up feeling rested and refreshed and, as you get older, you are likely to require less sleep. Some individuals seem to be able to manage on only four hours a night, while others complain that even with ten they still feel washed out.

Insomnia is not just being unable to sleep for as long as you want. Sleep may be very fitful causing you to wake feeling out of sorts and tired; you may take a long time to fall asleep, or may wake up in the early hours of the morning and be unable to fall asleep again. If you suffer from insomnia, try some of the following measures to alleviate the problem:

- take some exercise during the day, preferably in the fresh air, so that you feel tired at bedtime
- have a light meal early in the evening. If you eat a large meal within a couple of hours of going to bed, an active digestive system is likely to keep you awake
- don't drink a late cup of tea or coffee that contains the stimulant caffeine; have a decaffeinated or warm milky drink instead
- alcohol can interfere with sleep, so drink it only in moderation
- if you are working late, take at least an hour off to unwind before you go to bed
- have a warm bath to help you relax
- make sure the bedroom isn't too hot or too cold and if there is a background noise that you can't sleep through, such as traffic or music from next door, try using earplugs
- sleep on a firm but comfortable mattress
- get up at the same time each morning regardless of how well you slept
- if you are elderly, try having a short nap during the day – paradoxically, this may improve your night's sleep
- don't worry if you can't get to sleep: just resting in bed will be doing you some good
- at bedtime read for pleasure, not work or study.

See your doctor if your insomnia persists despite these measures. If you are under a lot of stress, or feeling anxious about something in your life, your doctor may recommend some form of muscle relaxation or breathing exercise to help you get off to sleep. Nowadays, you will normally be prescribed a sedative only as a last resort. A drug-induced sleep is not as restful and it is easy to become dependent on this type of drug, with unpleasant withdrawal symptoms if you stop it suddenly.

It may be that you need to take sleeping tablets for a few days to help you get back into your normal sleeping pattern if you are going through a particularly bad time. However, to avoid becoming dependent, it is best not to use sleeping tablets every night for longer than a week. Also, they tend to become less effective with regular use.

Irritable bowel syndrome

Irritable bowel syndrome is a disorder of the bowel muscle function. Although there is no specific physical abnormality, such as inflammation or an ulcer or tumour, this condition can produce distressing symptoms. Sufferers from an irritable bowel may complain of a wide variety of symptoms, ranging from colicky abdominal cramps, usually low down on the left side, excess gas, abdominal swelling and a bloated feeling and alternating bouts of diarrhoea and constipation, to nausea, vomiting, loss of appetite and extreme lethargy.

The recurrent abdominal pains are typically worse soon after eating a meal and ease off after passing wind or faeces.

As many as one in three of the population in the UK will suffer occasional symptoms of an irritable bowel (symptoms usually begin to cause problems between the ages of 15 and 40 years). One in ten people develops symptoms bad enough to consult a doctor.

Stress can certainly be one aggravating factor, but it is not the only cause. In fact, many men with irritable bowel syndrome have no problems with stress, anxiety or depression. When stress is playing a part, counselling and relaxation techniques can do more to relieve symptoms than any drug treatment.

Another important factor is diet. Some sufferers react badly to certain foods, such as wheat, dairy products and citrus fruits; simply identifying and avoiding these foods may be enough to ease the symptoms. About one-third of people with an irritable bowel benefit from slowly increasing their intake of high-fibre foods, such as fresh fruit and vegetables, wholegrain bread and cereals, rice and pulses. However, many others are made worse by this type of diet and should try a low-fibre diet.

It is also advisable to cut down on tea and coffee, but make sure you drink at least eight glasses of water each day, as fluids help maintain good bowel function. Take a laxative only if your doctor recommends one; in fact, an irritant laxative, such as senna, can make the pains worse.

See your doctor if you have persistent or recurrent symptoms; do not just assume you have this condition: a check-up is necessary to rule out more serious bowel disorders. You may be prescribed peppermint oil capsules or an antispasmodic drug to relax painful bowel muscle spasm, or a bulking laxative to soften and increase the volume of your stools.

Migraine

A typical migraine attack causes a throbbing headache, usually on one side of the head, with nausea and vomiting. Visual disturbances, such as seeing flashing lights or zigzag shapes, or partial loss of vision, may also occur, sometimes just before the onset of headache. Occasionally, an attack may cause numbness and tingling in the limbs and increased sensitivity to light and noise.

For many sufferers, a migraine attack can mean several hours of excruciating pain that makes it impossible to work or even think straight, followed by a day or more of feeling totally exhausted. Ordinary painrelievers often don't seem to help much, and the only solution is to retreat to a darkened room and try to sleep until the symptoms ease off.

Although the exact cause of migraine remains unknown, the throbbing headache is thought to be due to a temporary widening of blood vessels in the brain and scalp. Some people are able to identify and then avoid specific trigger factors that provoke an attack, such as missing a meal, sleeping in longer than usual, or eating a specific type of food over the previous two days.

Eating regularly, avoiding lying in (at the weekend or on holiday), and cutting out cheese, chocolate, oranges, peanut butter and certain alcoholic dri..ks such as red wine or spirits may help reduce the frequency of attacks. Unfortunately, however, the majority of migraine sufferers are unable to find such an easy solution.

If ordinary painrelievers, such as aspirin or paracetamol, on their own or combined with codeine, fail to improve your headache, an anti-inflammatory drug such as ibuprofen, which you can buy from the pharmacist, may help. Whatever brand of painreliever you use, it is important to take it as soon as you feel an attack coming on to get the best effect. Soluble or effervescent preparations are preferable because they work quicker.

See your doctor if you are suffering from frequent disabling attacks of migraine. You may be prescribed a preventive drug, such as a betablocker or sanomigran, which can stop migraine coming on but won't help an acute attack. However, although these drugs are often effective, they commonly cause side-effects – betablockers are associated with lethargy and sanomigran with weight gain. Sumatriptan, a new prescription drug taken by mouth or injection, can rapidly relieve migraine symptoms in most people.

Regular use of feverfew, a herbal preparation, has been shown to reduce the frequency of migraine attacks and decrease the severity of nausea and vomiting during an attack. Although you can grow your own feverfew plants, or buy feverfew tablets from a pharmacy or health store, it is best to consult a qualified herbal practitioner for advice on the correct dose for you.

A few people seem to be helped by acupuncture or hypnotherapy and, because stress can trigger migraine, it is worth trying relaxation exercises (see **Chapter 3**), which may help control attacks by reducing tension.

Myalgic encephalomyelitis (ME)

This mysterious disease, which usually strikes people in their late 20s or early 30s, is characterised by severe physical and mental exhaustion. Symptoms may include extreme muscle fatigue, muscle pains like hundreds of pinpricks, aching joints, headaches, disturbed sleep, loss of memory, difficulty concentrating, dizziness and blurred vision.

ME is also referred to as chronic fatigue syndrome, but it is more than just ordinary tiredness. During this illness, even the simplest activities, such as walking from room to room, require a tremendous effort. A typical description likens ME to having a severe bout of 'flu which seems to go on for ever. Symptoms can persist for several years, with intermittent periods of recovery interspersed with episodes of sudden relapse. However, most ME sufferers will make a full recovery eventually.

The exact cause is unknown, but experts believe that symptoms are brought on by an abnormal response to a viral infection, which in turn disrupts the function of the muscles and nerves. Many ME sufferers pinpoint the onset of their condition as a specific infection, usually of the throat or chest.

There is no conventional drug treatment for ME. Antidepressants were often prescribed in the past, but depression is thought to be a consequence rather than a cause of ME. Recovery from ME can be assisted and the chances of a relapse reduced by the following measures:

- drinking little or no alcohol
- cutting down on highly refined carbohydrate (sugary) foods
- avoiding extremes of temperature
- undergoing immunisation or a general anaesthetic only if essential
- taking an adequate period of complete rest
- gradually returning to normal activities over several months
- exercising gently and regularly, but never pushing yourself too hard.

Some ME sufferers are helped by alternative therapies such as homoeopathy, herbal medicine and aromatherapy. Recently, thermoregulatory hydrotherapy (TRHT), a technique in which the patient undergoes gradual immersion in cold water at a temperature of 16°C, has been shown to make a significant difference to symptoms after several weeks of daily exposure.

Obesity

The standard method used to define the terms overweight and obesity is to take the individual's body weight, measured in kilograms, and divide it by the square of his height in metres ($W \div H^2$). This formula produces a figure known as the body mass index (BMI – *see page 67*).

A man with a BMI between 25 and 30 is defined as being overweight, although occasionally this slightly higher than normal figure may be due to muscle bulk rather than fat. A BMI above 30 is defined as obesity.

In the UK, about ten per cent of men over the age of 40 are obese. The cause in most cases is a combination of overeating and not taking enough exercise to burn off excess calories. Your weight will remain stable only if your energy intake in the form of calories from food and drink is in balance with the energy expended to keep your body organs ticking over at rest, as well as fuelling your muscles when you exercise. Any excess supply of energy is converted into fat stores, which in men are mainly deposited around the abdomen as a paunch.

In addition to unhealthy eating and exercise habits, obesity also tends to run in families. If both your parents are or were obese, you stand a much greater chance of becoming obese yourself. However, this may not just be a genetic phenomenon, as an unhealthy lifestyle can also be passed on from one generation to the next.

A few men – the so-called 'underburners' – need fewer calories to satisfy their daily energy needs, and therefore have to be extra careful to keep their weight under control.

Older men are more vulnerable to becoming overweight or obese because their energy requirement gradually decreases. The loss of muscle tissue that occurs as a normal part of ageing means the body needs less energy for muscle cell metabolism at rest. Also, older men tend to take less physical exercise and therefore burn up fewer calories overall. Because it is difficult to change eating habits, the necessary gradual reduction in daily calorie intake to keep the balance between energy supply and demand is not made. As a result, fat will slowly build up and weight will steadily increase with advancing years.

Being overweight can be a serious hazard to your health. Not only will you tend to become tired and breathless more easily, but you will also be more vulnerable to a wide variety of medical disorders, including back pain, osteoarthritis, varicose veins, gallstones and even certain types of cancer, such as cancer of the colon, rectum and prostate. Obesity also increases the risk of high blood pressure, high blood cholesterol and diabetes, all of which are associated with a greater chance of suffering from a heart attack or stroke.

To prevent or control obesity, you need to pay attention to your diet and take regular exercise. Suitable diet and exercise programmes for men who are overweight are described in detail in **Chapter 2**.

Osteoarthritis

Osteoarthritis, the most common form of arthritis, is the result of wear and tear of the cartilage surfaces inside a joint causing pain, stiffness and swelling. This wearing out of the joint tends to occur gradually with advancing years. Most men in their 60s have osteoarthritis in at least some of their joints.

The joints most commonly affected are those that have taken the most punishment over the years – the hips, the knees and the joints at the base of the neck and lower back. Factors which increase the risk of osteoarthritis include being overweight, overuse of a joint playing a particular sport, or a serious or recurrent injury to a joint when younger.

There is no cure for osteoarthritis, but symptoms can usually be controlled with painrelievers, or anti-inflammatory drugs taken by mouth or applied to the affected joints as a gel. A doctor or physiotherapist may be able to recommend exercises to strengthen the muscles around an arthritic joint, which should also help to protect the joint against further damage.

In severe cases, where the arthritic joint has become very painful or stiff, sufferers may be referred to hospital for a joint-replacement operation.

Penis disorders

A wide variety of disorders can affect the penis. Penile warts, sexually transmitted diseases and the causes and treatment of impotence are discussed in detail in **Chapter 4**. Other penis disorders include:

Balanitis The glans (head) of the penis and foreskin become inflamed, resulting in a red, moist appearance with itching or discomfort. It is usually caused by infection, either with bacteria or a fungus such as thrush, and treatment is likely to be the appropriate antibiotic or antifungal drug prescribed by your doctor.

Poor hygiene may play a part in causing the infection, but thrush is invariably picked up during sexual intercourse with an infected partner, who should therefore be treated as well.

Having an abnormally tight foreskin (phimosis) which is difficult or impossible to pull back increases the risk of balanitis by preventing the man from washing under his foreskin properly. Most young boys have a tight foreskin, but this should not be forced back otherwise there is a risk that it will become damaged or stuck. Normally the foreskin becomes more mobile as the boy grows older, but if a phimosis persists and is causing either recurrent balanitis or pain during intercourse or masturbation, circumcision (*see over*) is usually recommended.

Occasionally, balanitis is due to irritation from residual laundry detergent on underpants, or an allergic reaction to a spermicide.

Priapism   This is a condition whereby erection becomes painful and abnormally prolonged in the absence of sexual arousal. It occurs when blood is unable to drain back out of the penis, for example, due to nerve damage, a blood clotting disease or blocked circulation due to infection. Nowadays, the most common cause is following self-injection therapy for the treatment of impotence (*see page 146*).

Emergency treatment of priapism is essential to avoid permanent damage. This may be by injection of local anaesthetic into the spine, or by withdrawal of blood from the penis using a sterile needle and syringe.

Peyronie's disease   Thickening of part of the fibrous sheath inside the penis causes it to bend at an alarming angle each time it becomes erect, making intercourse painful or impossible. This condition usually affects only men over the age of 40.

Although the exact cause of Peyronie's disease is unknown, it may be provoked by minor trauma to the penis during vigorous sexual activity. When the penis becomes flaccid, the thickened area may be felt as a firm nodule.

A few men require surgery to straighten the penis, which involves the insertion of special stitches on the opposite side to the bend.

Penile cancer   This extremely rare form of malignant tumour is more common in uncircumcised men and is associated with poor personal hygiene and smoking. The tumour usually first appears as a painless wart or a painful ulcer on the tip of the penis.

If diagnosed early, circumcision followed by radiotherapy may be successful without the need for further surgery. Therefore, always have an immediate check-up with your doctor if you develop any wart or ulcer on your penis that persists for over two weeks.

CIRCUMCISION

Surgical removal of the foreskin – circumcision – is a procedure in which the inner and outer layers of this flap of skin are cut away and the raw edges stitched together. This operation has been carried out for many centuries as a religious ritual on all male infants born into Jewish or Moslem families and by others for reasons of hygiene. Whereas in the past it would normally have been the rabbi or imam who performed the circumcision, it is now usually done by a surgeon, which should reduce the risk of complications, such as excessive bleeding or infection.

Nowadays, it is much less fashionable to circumcise boys purely for hygienic reasons because there is no reason why an uncircumcised man should not keep himself clean by pulling back his foreskin to wash away any build-up of secretions (smegma) each day.

Medical reasons for circumcision in adult men include an abnormally tight foreskin (phimosis), which is causing pain when the penis is erect or during intercourse, or recurrent infection under the foreskin – a condition known as balanitis (*see pages 216–7*).

In children and adults, circumcision is usually performed under a general anaesthetic. After the operation, intermittent application of an ice-pack may be recommended to reduce swelling and bruising. Also, a warm bath with a handful of table salt added to the water will help keep the wound clean. It may not be possible to wear underpants for a few days while the wound remains uncomfortable.

Peptic ulcer

The two main types of peptic ulcer are ulceration of the duodenum (duodenal ulcer or DU), which will develop in about one in ten people at some time in their lives, and a gastric (stomach) ulcer which occurs in about one in 30. Men are more likely to develop a duodenal ulcer than women, but the chances of a man or woman suffering from a gastric ulcer are about equal.

Both these forms of peptic ulcer usually first appear in middle age, but the peak age of onset for a DU is on average ten years earlier.

Typical symptoms of a peptic ulcer include a burning or gnawing pain in the abdomen, which will sometimes wake the sufferer at night.

While the pain from a DU is characteristically relieved by eating, only to reappear a few hours later, the pain due to a gastric ulcer is made worse by food and drink. Other symptoms that may occur with both types of ulcer are loss of appetite, nausea, vomiting, belching, feeling bloated and loss of weight.

Many ulcer sufferers only become aware of their condition if they develop a complication, such as severe abdominal pain due to the ulcer perforating, or if the ulcer bleeds, to cause vomiting of blood, or material which looks like coffee grounds, and the passing of black, tarry stools.

The ulcer may be diagnosed by gastroscopy, whereby a viewing instrument is passed through the mouth, down the oesophagus and into the stomach and duodenum. A barium X-ray examination, for which the patient drinks a solution of barium that shows up white on subsequent X-ray pictures, can also reveal both gastric and duodenal ulcers.

Thanks to advances in medical therapy, surgery for a peptic ulcer is usually reserved nowadays for those cases in which a complication has developed. In addition to antacids, which can relieve ulcer pain by decreasing stomach acidity, a range of powerful ulcer-healing drugs is now available.

A common problem, however, has been the large number of people who relapse within a year of their peptic ulcer being healed. One way to overcome this is to take a low dose of an ulcer-healing drug indefinitely.

A new approach has recently been introduced, which works on the basis that a particular type of bacterium found in the upper part of the digestive system is responsible for the formation of almost all duodenal ulcers. Eradication of these bacteria by taking a combination of two antibiotics and bismuth – a drug which also promotes ulcer healing – has been shown in trials to be highly effective at achieving a long-term cure.

To reduce your chance of developing a peptic ulcer, or suffering a recurrence once an ulcer has healed:

- stop smoking and cut down on alcohol, coffee and tea
- eat small meals at regular intervals and avoid a large meal within two hours of going to bed
- choose a painreliever that contains paracetamol, with or without codeine, rather than aspirin or any other type of anti-inflammatory drug.

Prostate enlargement

An enlarged prostate gland is a very common problem among older men. Because of the gland's position just underneath the bladder and surrounding the upper part of the urethra (the narrow tube that carries urine and semen to the tip of the penis), prostate enlargement may obstruct the normal flow of urine.

Each year in the UK about 350,000 men visit their GP because of urinary symptoms caused by an enlarged prostate, of whom one in ten needs surgery. In almost all cases, the cause is benign prostatic hyperplasia (BPH) – a non-cancerous condition.

While it is normal for the prostate gland to enlarge around the time of puberty, as part of male sexual development, why it should start growing again in so many men once they pass the age of 50 is not understood, although this renewed growth is known to be stimulated by male sex hormones produced by the testicles.

Characteristic symptoms of an enlarged prostate include:

- difficulty starting the flow of urine – you may have to push or strain
- a weak stream that may stop and start several times
- feeling that the bladder hasn't been completely emptied
- having to urinate again less than two hours later
- finding it difficult to postpone urination
- needing to urinate at intervals throughout the night, with consequent disruption of sleep
- dribbling after urination.

Embarrassment causes many men to delay seeing the doctor until their symptoms have become intolerable. However, treatment is usually successful at restoring near-normal urinary function.

To confirm that the prostate gland is enlarged, the doctor may perform a digital rectal examination, whereby a lubricated gloved finger is inserted into the rectum and the prostate palpated (felt) through the front wall of the rectum, which lies against the back of the gland.

The standard treatment for BPH is a surgical procedure called a trans-urethral resection of the prostate (TURP), in which a long narrow instrument (resectoscope) is passed up the urethra towards the bladder. At the tip of the resectoscope is an electrically heated wire loop that is used to shave away the obstructing prostate tissue, while the surgeon watches the procedure through a small telescope contained within the instrument.

TURP should make no difference to male libido, but it may occasionally cause impotence as a psychological response, particularly in men who haven't been properly counselled before their operation. A more common problem after TURP is retrograde (backward) ejaculation whereby, due to damage to an internal valve at the top of the urethra, semen is ejaculated back up into the bladder rather than out of the penis.

Retrograde ejaculation will cause the man to become infertile, although for most men old enough to require prostate surgery there is no desire to father a child. It should not make any difference to the enjoyment of sex, as long as both the man and his partner are aware of the reason why his orgasm is no longer producing a visible ejaculate.

New forms of treatment currently under investigation include the insertion of a tiny metal coil (stent) to open up the urethra inside the prostate, the use of a microwave beam to heat up and shrink the prostate, and a drug called finasteride which, by preventing hormonal stimulation of the prostate, also shrinks the gland and so improves urine flow. Another type of drug, which can help relieve prostate symptoms but doesn't alter the size of the gland, works by relaxing the smooth muscle inside the prostate. The resultant reduction of pressure on the urethra can make it easier to pass urine.

However, surgical treatment is still required in those men who have severe symptoms, or if complications have developed, such as recurrent urine infection, bladder stones, retention of urine in the bladder or kidney damage. Progress is now being made with the use of laser prostatectomy as an alternative to conventional TURP.

Self-help measures that may reduce symptoms in less serious cases of prostate enlargement include:

● restricting fluid intake after 6pm
● cutting down on alcohol and caffeine
● limiting spicy food, which can further irritate the bladder
● taking exercise during the day if your lifestyle tends to be sedentary.

Rheumatoid arthritis

Rheumatoid arthritis (RA) is a severe form of arthritis that affects roughly one million people in the UK. The exact cause of RA is unknown, but it is believed to be an auto-immune disease, in which the body's immune system starts to attack its own tissues, in this case the joints. Although RA may begin at any age, it most commonly strikes people in their forties. In some cases, infection by a virus is thought to be the precipitating factor.

Symptoms of RA include:

- pain, tenderness, swelling, redness and warmth, usually affecting several joints symmetrically on either side of the body
- joint stiffness, characteristically worse on waking
- weakness of grip in one or both hands
- sometimes fever, malaise, general muscle weakness and weight loss.

These symptoms tend to flare up intermittently, with long periods of remission in between which may last several months or even years. The diagnosis is made from a description of the symptoms and a physical examination of the inflamed joints. A blood test will usually show a high level of an abnormal protein known as rheumatoid factor.

Many RA sufferers only develop a mild disability and are able to remain mobile and independent. Treatment includes resting inflamed joints during a sudden flare-up, using splints, for example, and regular courses of physiotherapy at other times to loosen up the joints and strengthen the muscles that support them.

Non-steroidal anti-inflammatory drugs are prescribed to relieve the joint symptoms. In severe cases, drugs which slow down the disease and limit the amount of joint damage may be required – examples include gold salts, penicillamine and sulphasalazine – but all of these have potentially serious side-effects.

A variety of aids are available to help badly affected people overcome the disabling effects of RA, to cope with everyday tasks such as dressing and preparing food. Surgery may be necessary to correct a serious deformity, or to improve the range of movement in a joint.

Seasonal affective disorder

Seasonal affective disorder (SAD) is a type of depression that occurs during the winter months. In addition to making the sufferer feel low and miserable, possible symptoms include disturbed sleep, difficulty waking up in the morning or staying awake during the day, apathy, lethargy, fatigue, irritability, generalised aches and pains, reduced sex drive, loss of self- esteem and a craving for sugary foods which can lead to an unwanted increase in body weight.

As many as one in 20 people in the UK are thought to suffer from SAD each winter. The underlying cause is believed to be a biochemical imbalance in part of the brain known as the hypothalamus, brought on by a lack of exposure to natural sunlight.

If you have symptoms of SAD that have not been helped by spending more time exposed to natural daylight, then see your doctor. You may be referred to one of the specialist SAD clinics set up in different parts of the UK (contact SAD* for details).

Treatment, which is successful in the majority of SAD sufferers, involves phototherapy – exposure to a very bright ultraviolet light, emitted from a light box that is at least ten times more intense than normal domestic lighting, for up to four hours a day. Occasionally, antidepressants are also required.

Snoring

Snoring is the noise made by vibrations in the roof of your mouth. It occurs most commonly in those people who breathe through their mouth while they are asleep, although it is also possible to snore through your nose with your mouth tightly shut.

Any condition which blocks the flow of air through the nose may produce snoring, for example, a cold or sinus infection, a runny nose caused by allergy to dust, pollen or a particular food, polyps in one or both nostrils, a broken nose or enlarged adenoids. Your nose may also become blocked if the internal lining swells, which, apart from occurring as an allergic reaction, can happen as the result of stress, being overtired, smoking or eating a large meal.

Sleeping on your back increases the chance of snoring because this position encourages your tongue to slip to the back of your throat, partly blocking the air passages.

Simple home remedies for snoring include:

- losing excess weight
- sleeping in a more upright position, on pillows or by raising the head of the bed
- tying a scarf around the head and jaw to stop the mouth dropping open

- stitching a rolled-up sock or cotton reel to the back of the pyjama jacket (or nightgown) to make it too uncomfortable to sleep flat on your back
- putting a vaporiser in the bedroom, as a dry atmosphere encourages snoring
- cutting down on alcohol and not smoking
- avoiding late evening meals.

See your doctor if these measures don't make any difference, or if your snoring partner appears regularly to stop breathing during the night as well – a condition known as sleep apnoea. The doctor may recommend a plastic device, now available in most large pharmacies, which, by widening the upper part of the nostrils, can improve air flow and stop snoring. A neck collar can help some snorers by keeping their lower jaw held forward while they sleep.

A surgical operation may be necessary if the underlying cause is a nasal polyp, enlarged adenoids, or if the inside of the nose needs to be straightened. Steroid or decongestant nasal preparations may cure the problem if the nose becomes congested at night.

Stroke

The overall incidence of stroke each year in the UK is about 200 victims for every 100,000 people. Older people have a much greater chance of suffering a stroke, with half the cases occurring in the over-75s.

A stroke is caused by interruption of the normal blood supply to part of the brain, resulting in damage to those brain cells deprived of oxygen for more than a few minutes. The three main types of stroke are a cerebral thrombosis, in which a blood clot (thrombus) obstructs one of the main arteries in the brain; a cerebral embolism, whereby a fragment of blood clot that has broken off from elsewhere in the circulation blocks a brain artery; and a cerebral haemorrhage, caused by the rupturing of a blood vessel in the brain.

Symptoms of a stroke depend primarily on which part of the brain has been damaged, as each brain area controls specific functions related to particular parts of the body. Typical symptoms may include sudden onset of numbness or weakness, usually on one side of the body, loss of speech or slurring of words, a sudden severe headache, partial loss of vision, unexplained dizziness, confusion, a sudden fall or unconsciousness.

The diagnosis of a stroke is usually confirmed by a doctor carrying out a thorough physical examination. Occasionally, the extent of the brain damage may be assessed by a CT scan (a computer-generated cross-sectional X-ray) or some other brain-imaging technique.

If a stroke has been caused by a blood clot, drugs may be prescribed to dissolve the clot, to prevent the clot from enlarging, or to stop any further clots developing. A small daily dose of aspirin is commonly given to decrease the chance of a subsequent stroke. Only rarely is surgery performed to remove a blood clot or to stop bleeding from a ruptured artery.

The main element of stroke therapy is a rehabilitation programme that aims to improve physical abilities and restore independence. Although damaged nerve tissue will not regenerate, other parts of the brain may be trained to take over the functions of the damaged area.

Recovery is often a slow process and can be unpredictable. Although most of the improvement will occur in the initial few months, progress may continue to be made over several years. The success of stroke rehabilitation depends on the extent of brain damage, the skills of the various therapists involved, co-operation of family and friends and most importantly a positive attitude in the victim.

Measures to reduce the risk of stroke include:

- not smoking; limiting alcohol intake
- taking regular exercise
- eating a low-fat, high-fibre diet
- losing excess weight
- having regular blood pressure checks
- seeking medical attention if you suffer a TIA (*see below*).

TRANSIENT ISCHAEMIC ATTACK (TIA)

A TIA is a mini-stroke which causes symptoms similar to a normal stroke, but, because there is no permanent damage to the brain, these symptoms disappear completely within 24 hours, leaving behind no additional disability.

Typically, the victim of a TIA may suffer a sudden blackout, temporary loss of speech or vision, or transient loss of power or sensation in an arm or leg. Even though a full recovery may occur within minutes, it is still essential to see a doctor for a thorough check-up because a TIA is a warning signal that a major stroke could be on the way.

About ten per cent of strokes are preceded by one or more TIAs, with the time delay varying from a few days to several months. Tests will usually be carried out to check the circulation to the brain, for example, an ultrasound scan of the arteries, or angiography, in which X-rays of the arteries are taken after a dye is injected into the circulation. A CT scan (computer-generated cross-sectional X-ray) of the brain may be done to rule out other brain disorders such as a tumour.

For some people who have had a TIA, the doctor may recommend aspirin or anticoagulant therapy, or surgery to remove fatty deposits from one of the arteries supplying blood to the brain as a way of reducing the chance of a future stroke.

Subarachnoid haemorrhage
In this type of haemorrhage bleeding occurs over the surface of the brain between the middle and innermost membranes (meninges) that cover and protect the underlying nerve tissues. By contrast, when a stroke is caused by haemorrhage, the bleeding occurs within the brain itself.

Someone who suffers a subarachnoid haemorrhage typically develops a severe pain at the back of the head, which comes on suddenly and completely out of the blue, as if from a blow by a heavy object. The person will usually collapse and may lose consciousness for several hours or even days. The symptoms are similar to those of meningitis – headache, vomiting, neck stiffness, a dislike of bright light and drowsiness.

Generally, the bleeding occurs spontaneously from a blood vessel at the base of the brain, which has ballooned due to a weakness in the artery wall that has been present since birth. Only a few cases are brought on by a head injury or strenuous physical exercise.

Subarachnoid haemorrhage can happen at any age, but is most common between the ages of 35 and 60. Diagnosis is confirmed if blood is found in a sample of spinal fluid drained from the lower back, along with a CT scan of the brain to locate the bleeding. Initial treatment, apart from bed rest, may include a drug to lower abnormally high blood pressure and a drug to relax spasm in the brain arteries.

Angiography – an X-ray of the brain arteries taken after injecting a dye, which shows up white on the subsequent pictures – may be carried out to see if surgical repair is feasible. Depending on the type of blood vessel damage and the severity of the haemorrhage, an operation may be performed to open the skull and clip the leaking blood vessel.

Alternatively, the vessel may be sealed using a special glue or metal coil, positioned using the angiography catheter (tubing) that is fed into a blood vessel in the brain via an artery in the groin.

Although subarachnoid haemorrhage may prove fatal, either at the time of the initial attack or due to subsequent bleeding, many victims recover – some completely, others with a residual disability such as limb weakness, memory loss or recurrent seizures.

Testicular disorders

A wide variety of disorders may affect one or both testicles. Cancer of the testicle has been discussed earlier in this chapter (*see pages 188–9*). Some of the other more common testicular disorders are:

Undescended testicle   Occasionally, one or, even more rarely, both testicles fail to drop down into the scrotum. This condition occurs in about ten per cent of premature baby boys, but in only one per cent of boys born close to their expected date of delivery.

In many cases, the testicle descends on its own. However, if it doesn't come down within the first few months of life, surgical intervention is necessary. This operation, known as an orchidopexy, is usually performed before the age of five years to give the testicle a good chance of developing normally and also to reduce the risk of it failing to produce normal amounts of both sperm and testosterone in later life.

Retractile testicle   Another much more likely reason for one of the testicles appearing to be missing from the scrotum in a young boy is a condition known as a retractile testicle. Due to a powerful muscle reflex stimulated by cold or touch, the testicle is drawn up out of the scrotum into the groin. Careful examination by the doctor should distinguish a retractile from an undescended testicle.

Ectopic testicle   Here the testicle has migrated to an abnormal position, usually either in the groin or at the base of the penis, during development of the baby in his mother's womb. If this abnormality fails to correct itself spontaneously, surgery may be required to reposition the ectopic testicle in its rightful place.

Hydrocele   This is a collection of fluid in the scrotum which causes a soft painless swelling of the tissues surrounding one or both testicles. The cause in adults is usually unknown, although sometimes fluid is formed as the result of infection or injury.

Hydroceles occur most commonly in middle-aged men. Treatment is only necessary for a swelling large enough to be causing discomfort. Fluid may be drawn off using a sterile needle and syringe. However, if the hydrocele re-forms, surgery may be recommended.

Varicocele   The veins above the testicle, most commonly just the left one, swell up. A varicocele is caused by a damaged valve in the vein draining blood from the testicle. This disorder is thought to affect as many as 15 per cent of adult men.

The aching discomfort sometimes caused by a varicocele may be relieved by wearing underpants that provide better support for the testicles. Surgery, carried out through a small incision in the groin, is reserved for those men whose discomfort persists, or cases in which the varicocele is thought to be interfering with sperm production, thus causing infertility.

Epididymal cyst   This is a fluid-filled swelling, usually painless, on the epididymis, which is the long coiled tube lying against the upper back part of the testicle, where sperm matures. This type of cyst is common in men over the age of 40 and surgical removal is necessary only if it becomes tender or enlarged.

Spermatocele   This harmless sperm and fluid-filled swelling is also found on the epididymis. Again, surgical removal is necessary only if the swelling becomes large or uncomfortable.

Torsion of the testicle   Sudden severe pain and swelling of one of the testicles, sometimes with discolouration of the overlying scrotum and occasionally accompanied by abdominal pain and nausea, may be caused by the testicle twisting around in the scrotum, cutting off its blood supply.

Torsion occurs most commonly during puberty, although it can develop later. Emergency surgery is essential to prevent permanent damage to the testicle. The procedure involves untwisting the testicle and securing it in the scrotum with stitches.

If gangrene has already set in, the testicle will be removed, but as long as the other testicle is healthy, fertility should not be affected.

Orchitis   This inflammation of one or both testicles causes severe pain and swelling along with a fever. Orchitis may result from infection by the mumps virus, and about one-quarter of the few men who develop mumps after puberty suffer this complication.

Treatment is with painrelievers and icepacks, and symptoms usually settle down within a few days. Orchitis may cause the affected testicle to shrink, and can also interfere with fertility.

Epididymo-orchitis   In this condition, the testicle and its epididymis both become inflamed, usually due to a bacterial infection which in many cases has spread from the urinary tract. Symptoms include severe pain and swelling at the back of the testicle, accompanied by redness and swelling of the scrotum in some cases.

Because these symptoms can mimic a torsion of the testicle, surgical exploration may be necessary to confirm that the blood supply has not been obstructed. Treatment of epididymo-orchitis consists of bed rest and antibiotics. It may take several months for the testicle to return to its normal size.

GLOSSARY

acid reflux A backflow of stomach acids (which aid the digestion of food) into the oesophagus (gullet) causing heartburn. Acid reflux may occur when the muscular valve around the lower end of the oesophagus – which normally prevents these acids escaping from the stomach – is put under too much pressure, for example, from excess weight or from overeating. The cause may also be a weakness of this valve associated with a hiatus hernia (where part of the stomach protrudes upwards into the chest cavity through the diaphragm)

acute Sudden onset

addiction The need to use repeatedly a drug, such as nicotine, alcohol or heroin. Addiction (or dependence) can be physiological, in which case stopping the drug will cause unpleasant withdrawal symptoms, and/or psychological, with intense craving if the individual is deprived of the drug

adrenaline A hormone released by the adrenal glands in response to stress, fear, anxiety or exercise which stimulates a variety of changes inside the body, including an increase in the heart and breathing rates, diversion of blood from the digestive system to the muscles and a rise in blood sugar levels, all of which increase the body's physical efficiency

AIDS (Acquired Immune Deficiency Syndrome) A condition which develops as a result of infection with the Human Immunodeficiency Virus (HIV, *see below*). AIDS may result in a variety of diseases, most of which are due to the virus causing failure of the body's immune defences against infection and cancer

amino acids Chemical building blocks from which proteins are made that each contain carbon, nitrogen and oxygen. Each protein in the body contains up to 20 different amino acids linked together in long folded chains in a specific sequence

angioplasty A surgical technique to improve blood flow through an artery narrowed by disease. An inflatable balloon and/or powerful laser beam may be used to widen (or re-open) the narrowed (or blocked) section of the artery

antenatal Occurring before birth

antibiotic Any one of a variety of drugs that can kill or stop the growth and proliferation of bacteria inside the body. Originally derived from moulds and other living micro-organisms, nowadays the majority of antibiotics are made artificially from chemical ingredients

antibodies Proteins produced by lymphocytes (a type of white blood cell) in response to contact with an antigen (*see below*), which either neutralise the antigen or make it more vulnerable to destruction by other white blood cells

antigen Any substance recognised by the body as being foreign. An antigen causes the body's immune system to produce antibodies (*see above*) which neutralise or destroy it. Although antigens are usually proteins (such as parts of viruses, bacteria, fungi, pollen, dust mite faeces or a donated organ), other substances such as metal may have an antigenic effect by combining with and modifying one of the body's own proteins

antihistamine A type of drug which blocks some of the actions of histamine (a chemical which irritates and inflames tissues causing an allergic reaction, such as hay fever)

artery A tube with elastic, muscular walls which carries blood away from the heart

basal metabolic rate The amount of energy (Calories, *see below*) consumed by the body at rest to maintain vital functions such as heartbeat, breathing and digestion

betablocker A drug which prevents the stimulation of body organs, tissues and vessels both by sympathetic nerves and by adrenaline (*see above*) in the bloodstream. Betablockers may be prescribed to relieve symptoms of anxiety or an over-active thyroid gland, to prevent migraine attacks or angina, to lower high blood pressure, or to control abnormal heart rhythms

bile The thick greenish-brown fluid which is formed in the liver from broken-down red blood cells and other waste products; it is stored and concentrated in the gall bladder and released intermittently into the duodenum to help with the digestion of fats

blackhead A type of spot characteristically seen on the surface of the skin of acne sufferers

bypass surgery A procedure to restore the normal flow of blood, urine, intestinal contents or spinal fluid around a blockage which has developed in part of the body. Coronary artery bypass surgery – one of the most commonly performed bypass operations – is often effective in relieving angina or preventing a heart attack in men with obstructed arteries in their heart circulation

Calorie The unit used to measure the energy value of food and drinks. One Calorie (kilocalorie) represents the amount of heat required to raise the temperature of one kilogram of water by one degree centigrade

capillary The smallest type of blood vessel in the body. Networks of capillaries around the body receive blood from arteries and drain blood back into the veins. Because the capillary wall is only one cell thick it allows a free exchange of oxygen, nutrients, salts, water, carbon dioxide and other waste products between the bloodstream and surrounding tissues

carbohydrate The body's main source of food energy, carbohydrates are made up of saccharide molecules, which contain carbon, hydrogen and oxygen. Simple carbohydrates (sugars) cause a sharp rise in blood sugar and include sucrose (cane or beet sugar), fructose (fruit or honey sugar) and lactose (milk sugar). Complex carbohydrates (starches) have to be broken down before they can be absorbed, thus producing a steady, more prolonged rise in blood sugar levels. Starches are found in fruits, vegetables, wholegrain breads, cereals and pasta. A refined carbohydrate is one which has been processed, for example, white sugar or polished rice, lowering its fibre content and reducing slightly its vitamin and mineral levels

cartilage Dense connective tissue capable of withstanding considerable pressure. Different types of cartilage perform different functions throughout the body; elastic cartilage, for example, provides the framework for the outer part of the ear; disks of fibrous cartilage act as shock absorbers between the vertebrae and inside the knee

chemotherapy The use of one or more chemical substances to prevent or treat disease; the term is used most commonly to describe treatment prescribed to people with cancer, either to shrink a tumour or to reduce the chance of it spreading to other parts of the body

cholesterol A chemical found in the bloodstream and body tissues which is a key component of cell membranes and a vital ingredient of steroid hormones, including testosterone. Most cholesterol is produced by the liver when it processes digested saturated fat – only a small amount comes directly from cholesterol-containing foods such as eggs and some types of shellfish. Abnormally high amounts of cholesterol in the bloodstream increase the risk of a heart attack or stroke

chronic Persistent

cirrhosis   Scarring inside the liver as a result of its cells being damaged, for example, through excessive alcohol consumption or infection with hepatitis B

colitis   Inflammation of the colon, which may cause severe diarrhoea, blood or mucus in the faeces, pains in the lower abdomen and, sometimes, fever. Colitis may be due to a bacterial infection, amoebic dysentry or inflammatory bowel diseases, such as Crohn's disease or ulcerative colitis

colostomy   A surgical procedure whereby the cut end of the colon is brought through the muscles at the front of the abdominal wall to form a new opening (stoma) from which faeces can be evacuated into a disposable waterproof bag attached to the surrounding skin. A colostomy may be a temporary measure (to allow the bowel to heal after an operation) or a permanent one (if the rectum has had to be removed)

coronary thrombosis   A medical term for a heart attack in which one of the heart arteries is obstructed by a clot. This results in death of the heart muscle because it does not receive the vital oxygen and nutrients normally provided by the blood vessel) (*see also myocardial infarction*)

diuretic   A drug which increases the volume of water lost from the body in the urine. Diuretics may be prescribed to treat any disorder of the heart, kidneys or liver which has resulted in excessive fluid retention

ECG (electrocardiogram)   A recording of the electrical activity in the heart muscle associated with the contraction and relaxation of the atria and ventricles during each heartbeat. An ECG, which may be displayed on a monitor or traced out on a strip of paper, can be used to diagnose heart disease or to detect an abnormal heart rhythm

enzyme   A protein which speeds up a chemical reaction without itself being altered by that reaction; the many thousands of enzymes in the human body are essential for the cells, tissues and organs to survive and function normally

epididymis   The highly coiled tube (around seven metres long) at the back of each testicle which connects it to the vas deferens

expectorant   An ingredient found in some cough remedies which makes it easier to cough up sputum, usually by causing the secretions inside the airways to become thinner and less sticky

faeces   Waste material from the digestive tract which is normally eliminated from the body through the anus. Faeces consist of undigested food (mainly cellulose), bacteria (dead and alive), cells from the bowel lining, secretions from glands in the bowel lining, bile from the liver and water

fat   The most highly concentrated source of energy from food, each gram of fat provides around 38 Calories, about twice as much energy as a gram of carbohydrate. There are three types of fat – saturated, polyunsaturated and mono-unsaturated – which vary in their chemical composition and effects on the body. Saturated fats are found in animal and dairy products; polyunsaturated fats are extracted from plant seeds, for example, sunflower, safflower and soya bean; mono-unsaturated fats are found mainly in olives, peanuts and avocados. Too much of any type of fat increases the risk of obesity. However, saturated fat is also linked with heart disease because it increases the levels of cholesterol (*see above*) in the bloodstream

fibre   The indigestible parts of plant foods, such as grain husks, the skin and flesh of fruits and the tough fibrous material in vegetables. Although fibre has no nutritional or energy value, it is an essential ingredient in a healthy diet because it helps prevent constipation, regulates the absorption of sugar and digested fats, and can slightly lower blood cholesterol

gastritis   Inflammation of the stomach lining. In acute cases (*see above*) it may cause abdominal discomfort, nausea and vomiting and can be due to excessive alcohol consumption, aspirin usage or a viral infection. Chronic (*see above*) gastritis, as a result of, for example, smoking or alcohol abuse, may not cause any symptoms and may only be discovered during an investigation for some other disorder

haemoglobin   An iron-containing pigment (haem) combined with a protein (globin) which gives red blood cells their colour and enables them to pick up oxygen in the lungs and release oxygen as they pass through other parts of the body

haemophilia   An inherited blood-clotting disorder caused by an abnormal gene which results in a life-long tendency to bleed excessively following a minor injury, or to bleed spontaneously, for example, into joints or muscles. Treatment of haemophilia involves regular injections of the missing clotting factor obtained from donated blood

heart attack   *See coronary thrombosis and myocardial infarction*

hiatus hernia   *See acid reflux*

HIV-positive   Possessing antibodies to Human Immunodeficiency Virus in the blood. People who are HIV-positive are often completely free of symptoms of ill health; the average time for the infection to develop into full-blown AIDS is currently 8–10 years in the UK

hyperglycaemia   Abnormally high levels of sugar in the bloodstream, occurring in untreated diabetes or if a diabetic eats too many sugary foods and/or is not taking enough medication. Symptoms include drowsiness, acetone odour on the breath, confusion and, in severe cases, lapsing into a coma

hypertension   Abnormally high blood pressure

hypoglycaemia   Abnormally low levels of sugar in the bloodstream, most common in diabetics who have taken too high a dose of medication or too little carbohydrate food. Symptoms include nausea, dizziness, sweating, weakness, loss of co-ordination and confusion (*see also reactive hypoglycaemia*)

incontinence   Uncontrolled, unwanted loss of urine, much rarer in men than in women. In men, urinary incontinence is usually caused by obstruction of the normal urine outflow by an enlarged prostate gland. Incontinence of faeces, where a man becomes unable to control his bowel movements, is generally confined to older men and may be caused by severe or long-standing constipation

insulin   A hormone released into the bloodstream from the pancreas gland which stimulates the uptake of glucose (sugar) from the circulation into cells throughout the body and also influences the chemical processing of carbohydrates, fats and proteins. A deficiency or absence of insulin causes diabetes mellitus

keratin   A fibrous protein found in hair, nails and the outer layers of skin

lymph   Fluid within the lymphatic system

metabolism   The various chemical and physical processes occurring inside the body which result in energy production from nutrients (catabolism) and the growth and repair of tissues and organs from molecular building blocks (anabolism)

minerals   Chemical elements needed in the diet, usually only in small amounts, to maintain good health. Minerals known to play a key role in cell function include calcium, iron, potassium, sodium and zinc

mucus   A sticky fluid, produced by glands in the membranes lining many different parts of the body, which has a protective and lubricating function

myocardial infarction   A heart attack in which part of the heart muscle (myocardium) dies

neurosis   A mental illness where there is abnormal behaviour or thinking but where the individual remains in touch with reality and has some insight into his condition

nicotine   An addictive ingredient in tobacco which in small doses can have a slight stimulating effect on mood. Although not generally as harmful as some of the other toxic substances present within inhaled tobacco smoke, nicotine is likely to pose a health risk to people with high blood pressure or a circulation disorder because it causes narrowing of blood vessels

obesity   Excess fat. In men, such fat is usually accumulated as an abdominal paunch. A person with a body mass index (BMI – weight in kg divided by the square of the height in metres) of over 30 is considered obese

osteoporosis   Loss of bone substance causing the affected bones to become brittle and more vulnerable to fracture; it may be caused by poor diet, cigarette smoking, lack of exercise and high doses of steroids, and is much more common in women, particularly after the menopause, than in men

palpitation   The sensation of becoming aware of your own heartbeat, most often in a situation where the heart has started to beat faster and more powerfully than normal (although it can also occur where there is no change in the heart rhythm or rate). Palpitations which last longer than a few minutes or which are recurrent can be a symptom of anxiety, a heart disorder or an over-active thyroid gland

peptic ulcer   An erosion or crater in the lining of the duodenum, stomach or, more rarely, the oesophagus

peristalsis   Spontaneous rhythmical contraction and relaxation of the muscles in the walls of various hollow tubes in the body to produce a wave-like movement

postnatal   Occurring after birth

prostate gland   A gland about the size of a chestnut, situated just below the bladder and in front of the rectum, which contributes nutrients and enzymes to the seminal fluid

protein   An important nutrient, made up of thousands of chemical units known as amino acids (*see above*), which is obtained from animal and/or plant sources. The amino acids enable the body to make new proteins necessary for the growth, development, repair and maintenance of cells and tissues and the production of the various hormones and enzymes which regulate body function

psychosis   Severe mental illness which may involve delusions, hallucinations, disturbed thought processes, grossly abnormal behaviour and/or extreme alterations in mood. Psychosis differs from neurosis in that the sufferer loses contact with reality and lacks insight into the seriousness of his condition

psychosomatic illness   Any medical condition which may have been caused or made worse by psychological factors. It does not, as is often mistakenly thought, imply that the symptoms do not really exist, rather that an emotional factor, such as stress, may be a contributing factor

psychotherapy   The use of psychological methods to treat an emotional, behavioural or mental disorder. There are various types of psychotherapy, all of which are based on the therapist establishing a relationship with the individual which encourages personal development and better self-awareness, thereby helping the patient resolve his conflicts and difficulties

radiotherapy   The use of ionising radiation as a medical treatment, primarily used nowadays to shrink a cancerous tumour or reduce the chance of cancer spreading to other parts of the body

reactive hypoglycaemia   A rapid fall in blood sugar due to a sudden release of large amounts of insulin by the pancreas gland responding to the digestion of sugar-rich food. It can be avoided by sticking to snacks that contain starches, fats or proteins rather than sugars

Reference Nutrient Intake (RNI)   The quantity of a nutrient, such as vitamin C, which should be consumed each day to satisfy the nutritional needs of the average person (previously called the Recommended Daily Allowance)

saliva   A slightly alkaline watery fluid released into the mouth by the three pairs of surrounding salivary glands, saliva is the body's natural antibacterial mouthwash, which also acts as a lubricant to assist chewing and swallowing and dissolves chemical particles in food, allowing them to be tasted

sebum   An oily substance, released from the sebaceous glands within the skin, which helps keep the skin surface slightly moist and also has an antibacterial effect

semen   Creamy, sticky fluid, produced mainly by the prostate gland and seminal vesicles, which is forcefully released from the urethral opening at the tip of the penis during ejaculation and which contains fructose and a variety of other nutrients to help keep sperm alive

septum   Dividing wall between different areas of the body

sphincter   A ring of muscle surrounding a passage or opening in the body, contraction of which will partly or completely close off that area

237

sputum   Mucus produced by specialised cells within the lining of the bronchial airways which helps trap particles such as dust and smoke, thereby preventing them entering and damaging the lungs

suppository   Medication in a solid form suitable for insertion into the rectum, where it slowly dissolves and releases its ingredients. Some suppositories have a local effect, for example, to relieve constipation; others contain drugs which are absorbed into the general circulation to affect other parts of the body. They may be given to patients who have been vomiting to ensure the drug stays in the system

testosterone   The most important of the male sex hormones (produced mainly by the testicles, but also in small amounts by the adrenal glands), testosterone stimulates muscle and bone development and is responsible for the secondary sexual characteristics which start to appear in young men at puberty

tranquilliser   A drug which produces a calming effect. Minor tranquillisers (such as the benzodiazepines) are used to treat anxiety and other neuroses; major tranquillisers (such as the phenothiazines) are used to treat schizophrenia and other psychoses

trans-urethral resection of the prostate (TURP)   The commonest type of surgical operation for an enlarged prostate. A telescopic instrument is inserted into the urethra (under a general or spinal anaesthetic) and the obstruction cut away using an electrically heated wire loop

varicocele   A varicose vein surrounding the testicle, usually the one on the left side of the scrotum

vas deferens   A narrow tube that carries sperm from the epididymis at the back of the testicle to the urethra prior to ejaculation

venereal disease (VD)   An infectious disease spread by sexual intercourse (nowadays, more commonly referred to as a sexually transmitted disease)

vein   A vessel carrying blood towards the heart. Veins have much thinner and less elastic walls than arteries (*see above*) because they are under much less pressure

vitamins   Chemical compounds essential for health which cannot be made in the body, so must be obtained from the diet. The various roles of vitamins include stimulating the growth and repair of tissues, controlling chemical processes which release energy, and breaking down toxic substances which might otherwise cause cancer or heart disease

ADDRESSES

Acne Support Group
PO Box 230
Hayes
Middx UB4 9HW
(Write enclosing an s.a.e.)

Action for Victims of Medical
Accidents
Bank Chambers
1 London Road
London SE23 3TP
Tel 081–291 2793

ALANON
Tel 071–403 0888 (Mon–Fri,
10am–4pm)
*Helpline for family and friends of
recovering alcoholics*

Alcoholics Anonymous (AA)
General Service Office
PO Box 1
Stonebow House
Stonebow, York
N. Yorks YO1 2NJ
Tel (0904) 644026/7/8/9
Helpline 071–352 3001
(10am–10pm)

Alzheimer's Disease Society
Gordon House
10 Greencoat Place
London SW1P 1PH
Tel 071–306 0606

Arthritis Care
18 Stephenson Way
London NW1 2HD
Tel 071–916 1500
Freephone helpline on (0800) 289170
(Mon–Fri, 12 noon–4pm)

British Association of Cancer
United Patients (BACUP)
3 Bath Place
Rivington Street
London EC2A 3JR
Tel 071–613 2121 *advice and
counselling; freephone information service
for anyone outside the 071 area on*
(0800) 181199 (Mon–Thurs,
10am–7pm, Fri 10am–5.30pm)

British Association for Sexual and
Marital Therapy
PO Box 62
Sheffield
S. Yorks S10 3TS

British Cardiac Patients Association
(Zipper Club)
Belmont
30 Perne Road
Cambridge
Cambs CB1 3RT
Helpline (0223) 247431 (daily,
9am–7pm)

British Chiropody Association
The SMAE Institute
The New Hall
149 Bath Road
Maidenhead
Berks SL6 4LA
Tel (0628) 21100

British Colostomy Association
15 Station Road
Reading
Berks RG1 1LG
Tel (0734) 391537

British Digestive Foundation
PO Box 251
Edgware
Middx HA8 6HG

British Heart Foundation
14 Fitzhardinge Street
London W1H 4DH
Tel 071–935 0185

British Holistic Medical Association
179 Gloucester Place
London NW1 6DX
Tel 071–262 5299 (Tues,
12.30–6.30pm)

British Massage Therapy Council
c/o Shaun Doherty
3 Woodhouse Cliff
Headingley
Leeds
W. Yorks LS6 2HF
Tel (0532) 785601

British Migraine Association
178A High Road Byfleet
West Byfleet
Surrey KT14 7ED
Tel (0932) 352468

British Red Cross Society
9 Grosvenor Crescent
London SW1X 7EJ
Tel 071–235 5454

British Wheel of Yoga
1 Hamilton Place
Boston Road
Sleaford
Lincs NG34 7ES
Tel (0529) 306851

Brook Advisory Centres
National Office
153A East Street
London SE17 2SD
Tel 071–708 1390

CHILD
Suite 219, Caledonian House
98 The Centre
Feltham
Middx TW13 4BH
Tel 081–844 2468
(24-hour answer-machine
081–893 7110)

CRY-SIS Support Group
BM CRY-SIS
London WC1N 3XX
Tel 071–404 5011

Depressives Anonymous
(Fellowship of)
36 Chestnut Avenue
Beverley
N. Humberside HU17 9QU
Tel (0482) 860619

Depressives Associated
PO Box 1022
London SE1 7QB
Tel 081–760 0544 *(answer-machine)*

Diabetes Foundation
177A Tennison Road
London SE25 5NF
Tel 081–656 5467

Families Need Fathers
National Administration Centre
134 Curtain Road
London EC2A 3AR
Tel 071–613 5060

or BM Families
London WC1N 3XX
Tel 081–886 0970
*(Advice on ensuring that children
maintain a good relationship with both
parents when a couple split up)*

Family Heart Association
Wesley House
7 High Street
Kidlington
Oxon OX5 2DH
Tel (0865) 370292

Family Planning Association
27–35 Mortimer Street
London W1N 7RJ
Tel 071–636 7866

Gender Dysphoria Trust
International
BM Box 7624
London WC1N 3XX
Tel (0323) 641100

Group B Hepatitis Group
Flat 1
6 Southwell Gardens
London SW7 4SB
Tel 071–244 6514

Haemophilia Society
123 Westminster Bridge Road
London SE1 7HR
Tel 071–928 2020

Hairline International/
The Alopecia Patients' Society
Lyons Court
1668 High Street
Knowle
Solihull
W. Midlands B93 0LY
Tel (0564) 775281

Headway (National Head Injuries
Association)
7 King Edward Court
King Edward Street
Nottingham
Notts NG1 1EW
Tel (0602) 240800

Health Advice for Travellers
Helpline (0800) 555777

Hearing Concern
(British Association of the Hard of
Hearing)
7–11 Armstrong Road
London W3 7JL
Tel 081–743 1110

Herpes Association
41 North Road
London N7 9DP
Helpline 071–609 9061

Terrence Higgins Trust
52–54 Gray's Inn Road
London WC1X 8JU
Tel 071–831 0330
Helpline 071–242 1010 (daily, 12
noon–10pm)
Legal line 071-405 2381 (Wed,
7–9pm)

Human Fertilisation and
Embryology Authority
Paxton House
30 Artillery Lane
London E1 7LS
Tel 071–377 5077

International Glaucoma Association
(IGA)
Kings College Hospital
Denmark Hill
London SE5 9RS
Tel 071–737 3265

ISSUE (The National Fertility
Association)
509 Aldridge Road
Great Barr
Birmingham
W. Midlands B44 8NA
Tel 021–344 4414

M.E. Action Group
PO Box 1302
Wells
Somerset BA5 2WE
Tel (0749) 670799

Manic Depression Fellowship
8–10 High Street
Kingston-upon-Thames
Surrey KT2 6HP
Tel 081–974 6550

Migraine Trust
45 Great Ormond Street
London WC1N 3HZ
Tel 071–278 2676

MIND (National Association for
Mental Health)
Granta House
15–19 Broadway
Stratford
London E15 4BQ
Tel 081–519 2122

Myalgic Encephalomyelitis
Association
Stanhope House
Stanford-le-Hope
Essex SS17 0HA
Tel (0375) 642466
Helpline (0375) 361013 (Mon–Fri,
1.30–4pm)

National AIDS helpline
Tel (0800) 567123 *24-hour freephone*

National Association for Colitis and
Crohn's Disease
98A London Road
St Albans
Herts AL1 1NX
Tel (0727) 844296

National Association of Deafened
People
103 Heath Road
Widnes
Cheshire WA8 7NU
Tel 051–424 3977

National Asthma Campaign
Providence House
Providence Place
London N1 0NT
Tel 071–226 2260

National Back Pain Association
The Old Office Block
Elmtree Road
Teddington
Middx TW11 8TD
Tel 081–977 5474/5

National Eczema Society
4 Tavistock Place
London WC1H 9RA
Tel 071–388 4097

Psoriasis Association
7 Milton Street
Northampton
Northants NN2 7JG
Tel (0604) 711129

QUITLINE
Tel 071–487 3000
*(Counsellors offer advice to anyone
trying to stop smoking from
9.30am–10pm)*

Relate Marriage Guidance
Herbert Gray College
Little Church Street
Rugby
Warwicks CV21 3AP
Tel (0788) 573241

Release
388 Old Street
London EC1V 9LT
Advice line 071–729 9904
(10am–6pm)
('All-other-times' number 071–603
8654)

Repetitive Strain Injury Association
Chapel House
152 High Street
Yiewsley
West Drayton
Middx UB7 7BD
Tel (0895) 431134 (Mon–Fri,
2–4pm)

Royal National Institute for the
Blind (RNIB)
224 Great Portland Street
London W1N 6AA
Tel 071–388 1266

SAD (Seasonal Affective Disorder)
Association
PO Box 989
London SW7 2PZ
Tel (0604) 846070

Samaritans
General Office
10 The Grove
Slough
Berks SL1 1QP
Tel (0753) 532713

Society of Chiropodists
53 Wellbeck Street
London W1M 7HE
Tel 071–486 3381

Spinal Injuries Association
Newpoint House
76 St James's Lane
London N10 3DF
Tel 081–883 4296
*(Counselling available Mon, Wed and
Fri, 10am–4pm; Tues and Thurs,
4–8pm)*

St John Ambulance
1 Grosvenor Crescent
London SW1X 7EF
Tel 071–235 5231

Standing Conference on Drug
Abuse (SCODA)
Waterbridge House
32–6 Loman Street
London SE1 0EE
Tel 071–928 9500

Stroke Association
CHSA House
123–7 Whitecross Street
London EC1Y 8JJ
Tel 071–490 7999

Tenovus Cancer Information
Centre
142 Whitchurch Road
Cardiff
S. Glam CF4 3NA
Tel (0222) 619846
Freephone helpline (0800) 526527
(advice for patients and families
Mon–Fri, 9am–5pm; answer-machine
at other times)

Transcendental Meditation (TM)
Freepost WN5103F
Skelmersdale
Lancs WN8 6BR
Freephone (0800) 269303

TSHG (Transvestite Self-Help Group)
PO Box 3281
London E1 6JG
Tel 071–289 5240

Uncircumcising Information Resources Centre
PO Box 52138
Pacific Grove
California 93950
USA

Yoga for Health Foundation
Ickwell Bury
Biggleswade
Beds SG18 9EF
Tel (0767) 627271

BIBLIOGRAPHY

The following is a short list of books which offer further information on various topics covered within the text.

Zilbergeld, Dr B. 1980 *Men and Sex – A Guide to Sexual Fulfilment* (Fontana)

Masters, Dr W. & Johnson Dr V. 1966 *Human Sexual Response* (Little, Brown, out of print)

Lacroix, N. 1989 *Sensual Massage – An Intimate and Practical Guide to the Art of Touch* (Dorling Kindersley)

Isay, R. A. 1993 *Being Homosexual – Gay Men and Their Development* (Penguin)

Weeks, J. 1991 *Against Nature – Essays on History, Sexuality and Identity (Rivers Oram Press)*

Llewellyn-Jones, Dr D. 1991 *Everyman* (Oxford University Press)

Smith, Dr T. 1990 *British Medical Association Complete Family Health Encyclopaedia* (Dorling Kindersley)

Youngson, Dr R. M. 1992 *Collins Dictionary of Medicine* (HarperCollins)

Carroll Dr S. 1992 *The Complete Family Guide to Healthy Living* (Dorling Kindersley)

LaFavore, M. 1992 *Men's Health Advisor* (Rodale Press Inc.)

Pesman, P./*Esquire* Editors 1984 *How a Man Ages – Growing Older: What to Expect and What You Can Do About It* (Esquire Press)

Combes, G. & Schonveld, A. 1992 *Life Will Never Be The Same Again: Learning to be a First Time Parent* (Health Education Authority)

Braun, D. & Schonveld, A. 1993 *Approaching Parenthood Resource for Parent Education* (Health Education Authority)

Health Education Authority 1993 *A Complete Guide to Pregnancy, Childbirth and the First Few Weeks With a New Baby* (Health Education Authority)

Voluntary Agencies Directory 1993/4 (NVCO Publications, incorporating Bedford Square Press, 1993)

Wellings, K. et al 1993 *Sexual Behaviour in Britain* (Penguin)

INDEX

Other books from Consumers' Association

Preventing Heart Disease – Understanding and taking care of your heart

Caring for Parents in Later Life – The practical, financial, legal and emotional issues

Which? Medicine – The essential consumer guide to over 1,500 medicines in common use

Available from the *Which?* shop at 359–361 Euston Road, London NW1 (telephone: 071–830 7640); or by post from Consumers' Association, Castlemead, Gascoyne Way, Hertford X, SG14 1LH; or freephone (0800) 252100 for Access/Visa orders.

Free trial subscription to Which? way to Health

For positive advice on staying fit, a healthy diet or detecting health problems at an early stage, read *Which? way to Health*. Published every two months, it gives you the results of tests on health products, and practical advice to help you to take control of your own health and keep stress levels in check. *Which? way to Health* is truly independent: it takes no advertising, so it can tell you the things you want to know, not what advertisers want you to know. For details of our *free* trial subscription offer write to Dept. E6, Consumers' Association, FREEPOST, Hertford X, SG14 1LH.